# FOOD FO

# FOOD FOR VITALITY

Jonathan S. Christie, Ph.D.

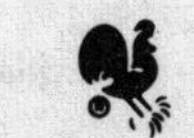

BANTAM BOOKS
TORONTO • NEW YORK • LONDON • SYDNEY • AUCKLAND

FOOD FOR VITALITY

A BANTAM BOOK 0 553 40347 8
First publication in Great Britain

PRINTING HISTORY
Bantam edition published 1992



This book is set in 10/12pt Sabon by
Kestrel Data, Exeter

Bantam Books are published by Transworld Publishers Ltd, 61-63 Uxbridge Road, Ealing, London W5 5SA, in Australia by Transworld Publishers (Australia) Pty. Ltd, 15-23 Helles Avenue, Moorebank, NSW 2170, and in New Zealand by Transworld Publishers (NZ) Ltd, 3 William Pickering Drive, Albany, Auckland.

Made and printed in Great Britain by
Cox & Wyman Ltd, Reading, Berks.

*For Maggie and everybody*

Everything should be made
as simple as possible,
but not simpler.
ALBERT EINSTEIN

The author wishes to make it clear that he is not a medical doctor. However, experts in this field frequently cannot agree. This book offers practical information to use in your quest for health, although no change of diet or exercise should be undertaken without consulting your doctor.

# *Acknowledgements*

So many people's efforts made this book possible that it is impossible to mention them all. However, without the researches of Dr Charles Bates, Dr Rodolfo Brenner, Dr Michael Crawford, Dr Max Gerson, Dr David Horrobin, Dr Donald Rudin, Dr Hugh Sinclair and others there would have been little to say.

Tracee Alexander, Peter and Sarah Bellwood, Dr Bernard Campbell, Dr John Douglass, Dr Michael Holden, Dr Arthur Janov, Sally Milow and Dr Michael Rosenbaum read and re-read the manuscript without complaint, and Wendy Campbell, Maggie Christie, Roger Hammond, Tony Mott and Annie Pinatelli provided needed encouragement. Thank you all.

# Acknowledgments

# *Contents*

# *List of Illustrations*

# *Foreword*

There are three pieces of the central enigma of man which when joined help give us a total picture of the workings of our neurophysiology. Candace Pert discovered our internal morphine system which controls the flow of information to consciousness. I believe that I have discovered the nature of the information repressed by Candace Pert's 'endorphines'. And Jonathan Christie has added the all-important dietary perspective to the solution of the puzzle of disease.

It seems that the much neglected essential fatty acids potentiate and modulate the actions of the repressive mechanisms, playing a significant role in mental ailments such as depression and premenstrual syndrome. An understanding of these acids allows us to strengthen our psychological defences without compromising our immune systems. This is an infinitely more natural approach than the alternative of painkillers and antidepressants.

The killer diseases of today, cancer, heart disease and diabetes, have an important dietary aspect which cannot be neglected, and no treatment can be considered complete without proper nutrition. And it is clear that in health, one will not feel one's best when essential nutritional elements are deficient.

We learn in this book that even though our diets may not be deficient in essential fatty acids, other dietary shortcomings can prevent our bodies making use of them. For example, eating saturated fats present in foods such as beef, dairy products and margarines compromises the essential fatty acid metabolism. This predisposes to the typical Western diseases such as heart afflictions, cancer and arthritis. There are psychological correlates to these deficiencies such as Seasonal Affective Disorder, manic depression and obsessional states.

The point of this book is a chance at better living through something as ordinary as eating. It is simply a logical approach to what we do all the time. It is exciting because it offers answers to serious problems heretofore considered almost refractory to treatment.

*Dr Arthur Janov*
*The Primal Training Center*
*1205 Abbot Kinney Boulevard*
*Venice, CA 90291, USA*

# *Introduction*

Far too many of us have trouble coping with the everyday stresses of modern life. Traffic jams and office pressures make us tense and irritable. Long commutes and working hours leave us little time or energy for exercise. Business lunches and working snacks play havoc with complicated diet plans. And weekends are too often used to catch up on our backlog of work, or to collapse in front of the television with a drink and a snack in an effort to unwind.

We mean well, and worry more about our health as we get older. But it's hard to translate good intentions into action, and we put off doing something from day to day. After all, we're not suffering from a serious disease – at least, not *yet*.

Instead, we end up tired, a little overweight, sometimes depressed and irritable, with a cholesterol level that's a bit too high and maybe a tendency to overdo the alcohol occasionally. We're not exactly ill, but we're not exactly well, either, and the quality of our life is not all it should be. With so many women in the work force these days, this is a problem which affects everybody. Perhaps most of all the working mother who's trying to hold down two jobs at once.

In fact, fatigue is such a universal affliction that it's mentioned in more than three-quarters of all doctor visits. As a Marriage, Family and Child Counsellor, I saw how bad moods, depression and irritability can cause marriages to fail, and how psychotherapy can address only part of the problem. However, as a suddenly diabetic adult, I learned at first hand how simple dietary changes can radically improve mood and energy levels as well as solve mysterious health problems, and also lessen cravings for 'the wrong stuff' – alcohol, cigarettes and junk food. After all, the body affects the mind as well as vice-versa.

The key to these beneficial effects lies in revolutionary new research into the role of dietary fats in the regulation of virtually every function of the human body. It's now known that not all fats are bad for you. There are 'good' fats, called omega-3 and omega-6 oils, found in fish and vegetable oils among other foods. These fats are called 'essential' because they are literally essential for health. This is because they are part of the structure of every cell of the body, because they are vital for brain and blood vessel function, because they are needed for transporting cholesterol and because *prostaglandins* are created from them.

Prostaglandins are short-lived, hormone-like chemicals made by every cell of the body to control a very large variety of metabolic processes, including immune response, blood pressure, cholesterol level, brain function, inflammation and allergic responses. New functions are being discovered daily, and the research on prostaglandins and health is considered so important that the 1982 Nobel Prize for Medicine was awarded to scientists working in this field.

Research has linked disordered *essential fatty acids* and prostaglandins with an impressive list of conditions, including heart disease, cancer, overweight, susceptibility to stress, premenstrual tension, depression, alcohol dependence, hypertension, impaired immunity, asthma, eczema, high cholesterol and even hyperactivity in children.

Hence, it's likely that a new deficiency disease syndrome has been discovered, and that the essential fatty acids from which prostaglandins are made will soon come to take their place beside vitamins and minerals, many of which are themselves turning out to be essential partly because of their roles in the essential fatty acid prostaglandin metabolism.

Studies involving dietary strategies for correcting the prostaglandins have reported weight loss, healthier skin, stronger nails, more restful sleep, more rapid recovery after exercise, less premenstrual tension and greater tolerance for, yet less need of, alcohol. These studies have also consistently reported, almost as side-effects, increased energy and self-esteem with less irritability and depression.

Two recent studies revealed connections between emotional states and heart disease. The first found that one third of heart patients were deeply depressed[1], the second that hostility boosts the risk of death from all causes, and especially from heart attacks[2]. For years, some researchers believed that an aggressive 'Type A'* attitude promoted heart disease. Now, however, it seems likely that there's a third factor which is the real cause of hostility, depression and heart attacks – disordered prostaglandins. Combining this new essential fatty acid and prostaglandin research with the known benefits of eating unrefined foods creates a way of eating which, remarkably, controls the emotions. People feel profoundly *better* eating this way.

This may be because we have strayed so far from our hereditary diet. This interesting idea stems from the work of Dr Charles Bates of Canada, who became intrigued by the considerable increase in disease among coastal Vancouver Indian communities who switched from their traditional, salmon-based diet to a Western diet. Using sophisticated blood tests, Bates found that the Indians developed essential fatty acid disturbances on the Western diet. He concluded that, because of their genetic adaptation, *they must stay close to their hereditary diet if they are to remain healthy.*

Most people in England have a northern coastal ancestry which includes some Scots, Welsh, Irish or Scandinavian blood. Emerging research suggests that these races ate fish-centered diets with whole grains for so many thousands of years that they cannot cope well without them now. The typical modern diet, low in essential fatty acids, disrupts the prostaglandin metabolism of such people, predisposing them to obesity, diabetes, rheumatoid arthritis, heart attacks, alcoholism and even schizophrenia.

Those without such hereditary weakness are by no means out of danger, since poor food choices can negate even a strong prostaglandin metabolism, and *everybody's* prostaglandin metabolism weakens with age, regardless of race. However, we who eat a Western diet can prevent the senseless, painful and *self-inflicted* deterioration from which we suffer with simple steps.

*Highly competitive behaviour such as working compulsively to meet deadlines.

# *1: Live Long And Prosper With The Essential Fatty Acids*

***Men occasionally stumble over the truth, but most pick themselves up and hurry off as though nothing had happened.***

WINSTON CHURCHILL

In the hectic modern world in which we all live, the one commodity in the shortest supply for all of us is time – time for contemplation, to stop and smell the roses, go for a drive, play with our children, walk in the country, see a film, read a book, or simply lie in a deck chair and think.

But even our thinking processes are conditioned by the speed at which things move these days. When I used to set aside time to relax, sooner or later I'd find myself making frantic mental lists of things I should be doing: mend the fence, fix the lawn mower, wash the car, return my phone calls, get my wife some flowers – plus three constant items which always appeared: LOSE WEIGHT. EAT A HEALTHIER DIET. TAKE LIFE MORE CALMLY.

One day, I was chatting about this with my neighbours Nick Travis and Laura Thomas. They laughed out loud, recognizing at once a similarity between their mental lists and mine – at least in respect of those last three items.

Nick is 45, a harried, mid-level advertising executive. He's conscientious, hard-working, overloaded and somewhat compulsive. Divorced from his wife, who moved to the country with their two children, he manages to see them every other weekend, an arrangement he finds totally inadequate.

Although outwardly calm, he often seethes with fury inside

when events seem to conspire against him. His keen sense of humour carries him through many of the petty crises of the day, but he can't get rid of his underlying tension. He doesn't broadcast it, but he doesn't feel good – and secretly, it scares him.

Following a day's work, he's often so tired that he needs at least a couple of drinks before he can even start to unwind, staring at the TV with glazed eyes before falling into bed around eleven o'clock.

Laura is 41, a successful commercial artist with two children from her former marriage, proud that she's holding down a well-paid job as well as being a good mother. She met Nick at a tennis tournament and moved in with him five months later. They enjoy each other's company, and Nick likes her kids and they all go camping once a year. Laura still has fantasies of quitting her job and painting full time.

Every month, she suffers from severe premenstrual tension. She has food allergies and a tendency towards depression. She struggles hard to stay cheerful, and Nick always lends her a sympathetic ear and a shoulder to cry on. But occasionally her children irritate her so much that she loses her temper in spite of herself, and then spends days gripped by remorse.

Deep down, both Nick and Laura admit to feelings of powerlessness when confronted by the three constant items on their mental lists – as Nick says, New Year's resolutions that are never fulfilled and run on year to year: LOSE WEIGHT. EAT A HEALTHIER DIET. TAKE LIFE MORE CALMLY.

To them, as to most of us, permanent weight loss is an impossible dream because a healthier diet requires an effort far beyond their available will-power. Winning the Pools seems like the only thing that might improve their mood.

In recent months, both of them have re-dedicated themselves and started to eat more carefully. Laura wants to trim down her figure and feel better about herself. Nick has reacted badly to the early death of a couple of friends from college. He wants to eliminate his severe bouts of indigestion and head off a possible heart attack – which killed both his father and grandfather. Despite their efforts, both remain steadfastly overweight and experience great difficulty in controlling their appetites when eating away from home, as their jobs often force them to do.

So the trio of resolutions remain unfulfilled – LOSE WEIGHT. EAT A HEALTHIER DIET. TAKE THINGS MORE CALMLY. The good news is, there's a simple way to accomplish all three objectives!

## *The Cavalry Is Coming*

Nick and Laura are typical. They are two of the nicest people you could hope to meet, anxious to improve themselves in any way they can. But, despite their material success, why do they feel stressed, moody and dissatisfied so much of the time? The answer is this: both have symptoms typical of a widespread and insidious condition, mild *functional** deficiencies of the essential fatty acids. I'll explain what this means shortly. For now, let me tell you what correcting this problem can do for them.

Nick's fatigue will lift, his desire for alcohol will lessen and his hangovers will be less severe. His cholesterol level and blood pressure will decrease, and his heart attack risk will fall.

Laura will find that almost all symptoms of her PMT will be controlled, and her food allergies will also improve. Incredibly, their appetites will become easier to control, especially if they avoid certain 'trigger' foods such as coffee. Without any heroic, superhuman measures, their overweight will slowly melt away.

Most amazing of all, Nick's concealed fury and Laura's depression, irritability and hair-trigger temper will become rare exceptions instead of everyday events. This means that they'll spend less energy controlling unfortunate impulses and maintaining a positive attitude by sheer effort of will. The effect will be a lifting of fatigue, a surge of energy which begets optimism and allows more grace under pressure.

This might seem difficult to believe. However, it happens all the time, but mostly for people who are very persistent. One woman whose PMT made her life a misery consulted no less than *sixteen* health professionals before she found the answer. Her 'bad days' decreased from two weeks to two days before her period after she switched to the way of eating that I'm proposing in this book.

*This medical term means there's nothing physically wrong, and there's probably no shortage of essential fatty acids in Nick and Laura's diet.

It sounds too good to be true, but the suggestions which follow come from the laboratories of reputable scientists, and many have been proved effective in clinical trials. This knowledge is just beginning to percolate through to health professionals, but there's no reason why Nick, Laura or you should have to wait for this process. No outlandish foods or bizarre, impossible diets are involved, merely a shift in emphasis. Here's how it works:

## *Essential Fatty Acids to the Rescue*

Much of this book is about the benefits of eating the right oils and the nutrients which help the body metabolize them. *Not all fats are villains*, and it seems that certain oils are vital for both physical and mental health. These oils are called 'essential' because, like vitamins, our bodies can't make them and we must obtain them from food. Chemically speaking, they're acids. Hence, they're called *essential fatty acids**.

Eskimos, for example, eat about the same amount of fat and cholesterol as in the UK diet, yet their rate of heart attacks is very low. One difference is that the Eskimo diet contains about twenty times more of the essential fatty acids derived from fish oil than our diet. Their experience tells us that it's not primarily the *amount* but rather the *types* of fat we eat which cause our problems.

The wrong kind of fats may make appetite difficult to control, so that overweight and a host of maladies may result. On the other hand, dozens of seemingly unrelated afflictions like high cholesterol, hypertension, low resistance to infections, arthritis, allergies and bad reactions to foods have responded to measures which restore the essential fatty acid metabolism. There's even evidence that the essential fatty acids help the body to fight cancer!

Other symptoms of functional essential fatty acid deficiencies include fatigue and a fundamental pessimism which sours the enjoyment of life. Alcohol provides relief partly by temporarily

*Fatty acids are the building blocks from which fats and oils are made. Fatty acids may be saturated (these predominate in meat and dairy products), mono-unsaturated (olive oil, avocado) or polyunsaturated (as in safflower oil). The essential fatty acids are both polyunsaturated. All fats and oils contain these three types of fatty acids; it's their proportions which matter.

reversing deficiency effects, but may consequently become impossible to resist. A hair-trigger temper, digestive difficulties and depression can complicate the picture further.

If you suffer from these conditions, you may put them down to stress, but this merely answers a question with a riddle: why are some people able to withstand enormous stress with a sunny disposition while others crumble under far smaller loads? I believe that the answer lies in their diets.

Fatigue, depression, irritability and overweight affect a very high proportion of people, and far too many of us die from heart disease. New research suggests these conditions are related, and that functional shortages of essential fatty acids contribute to them all. Furthermore, these symptoms often occur together. The two studies mentioned in the Introduction found that heart attack victims were very likely to be depressed, and that doctors and lawyers who had been overly hostile as students were far more likely to die (especially from heart attacks) in the next twenty-five years. Further, at least two studies have found that depression increased the risk of dying of cancer[1]. These 'symptom clusters' may occur because these difficulties are all caused by the same thing. Thus, *both depression and the hostile 'Type A' behaviour thought to cause heart attacks may simply be functional essential fatty acid deficiency effects, like the heart attacks themselves.*

Nuisance problems caused by functional essential fatty acid deficiency include unhealthy skin (dandruff, flaking, itching and dryness), brittle nails, lumpy breasts prone to premenstrual tenderness, dry eyes (often experienced as a tired, prickly feeling while driving or watching TV), dry mouth, food allergies and food cravings, an oily complexion and 'atopy'.

Atopy is the name for a surprisingly widespread inherited condition which predisposes to allergies, including atopic eczema, hay fever, asthma and even some migraine headaches*. In atopic families, various members may suffer from different conditions, or even from several conditions at once. Nearly three-quarters of hyperactive children[2] and Chronic Fatigue Syndrome sufferers[3],

*One study found that 80% of all colds were caught by atopic individuals (Arthur F. Coca, M.D., *Familial Nonreaginінc Food Allergy*, Thomas, Springfield Il., 1945).

and more than three-quarters of women who suffer from premenstrual tension[4] are atopic. It may be that atopy is caused by a family's diet being functionally deficient* in the essential fatty acids over several generations[5]**, *since recent experiments with rats indicate that essential fatty acid-rich diets, once started, improve health progressively for three and four generations*[6]. Thus, a mother's deficiencies may degrade the health of her babies so seriously that their offspring cannot achieve optimum health for *several generations*, however good their diet.

Serious conditions involving disturbed essential fatty acids include high cholesterol and heart disease, cancer, multiple sclerosis, cystic fibrosis, susceptibility to stress, over-reliance on alcohol, overweight and obesity, rheumatoid arthritis, bad temper, premature ageing and senility, depression, 'winter depression'***, carbohydrate craving and premenstrual tension. If, like Nick and Laura, you or someone close to you suffers from any of these difficulties, this book can help.

## This Is a Time of Opportunity

***A new scientific truth does not triumph by convincing its opponents and making them see the light, but rather because its opponents eventually die out, and a new generation grows up that is familiar with it.***

MAX PLANCK, ORIGINATOR OF THE QUANTUM THEORY (*1858–1947*)

Medical practice and dietary recommendations always lag behind research. This is as it should be. To avoid mistakes, there must be clinical trials before we adopt new ideas.

*A '*functional deficiency*' means the diet contains either too much total fat, too much oil altered by processing as in margarine, or low levels of certain vitamins and minerals the body needs to process fats and oils. *Actual* dietary essential fatty acid deficiency probably occurs only rarely.

**Breast-feeding is powerfully protective against the development of atopy. One symptom of EFA deficiency is increased permeability of the skin, including the lining of the intestines, so bottle-feeding exposes the infant to milk antigens very early in life. Another EFA deficiency symptom is poor T suppressor cell function, which causes an overactive immune system. Hence bottle-feeding may be the precipitating factor in the development of atopy.

***Also known as Seasonal Affective Disorder.

However, every now and again, there comes a time when research from different fields converges, creating a new way of looking at the relationship between diet and distress. At such times, there is an opportunity to leapfrog the lengthy process of experimental validation, by-passing the intellectual inertia which slows the adoption of new ideas.

In 1747, for example, Surgeon's Mate James Lind proved that citrus juice both prevented and cured scurvy, the vitamin C-deficiency disease which decimated ships' crews on lengthy voyages. It was not until 1795, however, that the Admiralty adopted daily doses of prophylactic citrus juice, and British sailors there- after became known as 'limeys'. During the forty-eight years that elapsed between Lind's discovery and the Admiralty's action, more than 100,000 British sailors died needlessly of scurvy!

Incredibly, it had been known for a century or more that scurvy grass (watercress) *prevented* scurvy, but, by an almost inconceivable failure of imagination, nobody thought to use it in order to *cure* the disease.

Similar tales exist for beriberi and thiamine, pellagra and niacin, pernicious anaemia and vitamin $B_{12}$ and rickets and vitamin D. In every case, the idea of a dietary deficiency was pooh-poohed initially because conventional wisdom attributed the causes of these diseases to Pasteur's infectious agents, the germs*. Since no treatments were available during the years between the discovery and acceptance of their causes, untold numbers of people were harmed in the meantime. *However, the better informed were able to change their diets to include more unrefined foods in advance of public health recommendations, and were protected.*

Today, history is repeating itself. It's likely that a new deficiency disease syndrome has been discovered, and that essential fatty acids will soon be as well-known as vitamins. For one thing, essential fatty acid derivatives are apparently vital to the body's communications system – and just as modern society might falter and collapse without the telephone service (which conveys everything from state secrets to bank balances, as well as casual

*Oliver Wendell Holmes, an American doctor who died in 1904, wrote that 'It is so hard to get anything out of the dead hand of medical tradition.'

conversation), so the body is plunged into chaos when the essential fatty acids are out of balance.

Much research suggests that simple dietary changes will lessen the risk of heart disease and cancer, and improve chronic discomforts like irritability, rheumatoid arthritis, depression and premenstrual tension. These changes will also alleviate a host of 'minor' conditions that may never reach a doctor's office, but which nonetheless make life miserable.

The essential fatty acids' panacea-like effects are the very opposite of what modern medicine deems respectable. The notion of a single remedy for many diseases is often looked on as the stuff of quackery. Despite this, it appears that faulty essential fatty acid metabolism is involved in literally *hundreds* of diseases, including mood disorders such as depression, irritability, and even schizophrenia and manic depression. My own experience confirms this. Before I began experimenting with essential fatty acid-rich diets, I had days of fierce exhilaration, and other days of profound melancholy. Sometimes I felt so irritable that I erupted at the slightest thing. Once I started eating the right foods, I found that my mood swings were largely replaced by a wonderful new sense of calm. I even found that I could practically choose my mood a few days in advance just by changing what I ate!

## Exciting New Developments

Recent prostaglandin research discloses ever more amazing potential benefits from fish oils. For example, in gerontology (the study of the aged), it's well-accepted that low-calorie diets are the only way to extend life. The explanation is probably that a low-fat, low-calorie diet increases the activity of the essential fatty acid-to-prostaglandin pathway by up to three times, boosting levels of the protective prostaglandins – which probably also accounts for Nathan Pritikin's famous success with heart patients. In the Pritikin Program, heart patients on very low-fat diets are put on quite strenuous exercise, the kind of activity which cardiologists used to say would guarantee another heart attack. Far from coming to harm, most make full recoveries, although the low levels of essential fatty acids in the Pritikin diet do eventually cause trouble as detailed by Pritikin's former Director of Nutrition, Anne Louise Gittleman, in her book *Beyond Pritikin**.

All the same, gerontologists were surprised when a study showed that mice fed certain unlimited diets actually lived longer than low-calorie mice[7]. The only unlimited diets which had this effect contained fish oils carefully protected against oxidation, and the mice maintained a youthful appearance until very late in their lives**. Even though the mice were of a strain which develops rheumatoid arthritis and kidney decline in later life – just like people – the fish-oil group were as free of these conditions as the low-calorie mice, and had the lowest cholesterol levels of all the groups!

In another study, a strain of rats prone to high blood pressure were protected by an essential fatty acid-rich diet, and *the benefit increased to the third and fourth generation*[8]. This has the exciting implications that our health may depend in part on what our parents ate, and we may be able to do great things for the health of our unborn children just by eating the right food.

This research also corroborates the conclusions of Dr Weston Price, an American dentist who travelled the world in the thirties, searching for people with perfect teeth. Price found that those on primitive diets, wherever he found them, had excellent teeth, outstanding general health and sunny dispositions. Incredibly, he found that most primitive cultures went to great pains to make sure their mothers-to-be were properly nourished, reserving for them such extra-rich foods as salmon roe. Using taboos and social restrictions, some cultures made certain that babies were spaced several years apart, ensuring they were born to mothers who were not nutritionally depleted. Scientists have recently discovered that this practice minimizes birth defects. For all our technical sophistication, we're only now beginning to appreciate the nutritional wisdom these cultures accumulated from their collective experience.

Research suggests that essential fatty acids are fully capable of

*Bantam, London, 1988

**Rodents' essential fatty acid requirements are significantly different from those of humans, but this study is exciting nonetheless because it suggests the auto-immune diseases may respond to dietary changes.

preventing many of the diseases of old age which we take for granted. If these effects hold true for people – and there's no reason to suspect they won't – we can expect an extended, productive middle age followed by a brief decline, changes which will transform the very nature of our society.

## *Your Hereditary Diet*

Canadian psychologist Dr Charles Bates has pointed out that some races are much more prone to nutritional deficiencies than others. Bates became intrigued by the vast increase of health problems such as overweight and rheumatoid arthritis which occur in coastal Vancouver Indian communities who switch from their traditional, salmon-based diet to a Western diet. Through sophisticated blood tests, he found the Indians were developing deficiencies of essential fatty acid derivatives on Western foods, and that *their genetic adaptation made it inevitable that their health would fail unless they ate their hereditary diet**.

If any of your ancestors came from a northern coastal region such as Scandinavia or Scotland, they got plenty of the essential fatty acid derivatives necessary for health ready-made**. Therefore, their essential fatty acid enzyme pathways (the cellular 'production lines' for converting essential fatty acids into derivatives useful to the body) didn't need to be as strong as those of inland hunter-gatherers, who had to make their derivatives from scratch.

It is entirely possible that a fragile essential fatty acid enzyme pathway combined with the wrong diet can lay you open to all the problems which may be caused by functional essential fatty acid deficiencies, including depression, irritability and alcoholism.

The racial groups popularly stereotyped as being fond of alcohol, such as the Scots, Scandinavians, Irish and American Indians, are particularly vulnerable. As little as 25% ancestry from such a group can bind you to inflexible dietary requirements,

*The Indians lack essential-fatty-acid-processing enzymes not needed on their EFA-derivative-containing traditional diet.

**In fish, animal organ meats such as liver, seeds and whole grains. Haggis, for example, contains oats and sheep offal.

with devastating consequences if these requirements aren't met. The typecast alcoholic Irishman, red-nosed Scot and hard-drinking, suicidal Scandinavian may exist because of genetic enzyme weaknesses combined with modern diets radically different from those eaten during the evolution of these races.

Almost everybody in the UK shares ancestry with a vulnerable racial group. And even if you are not at risk because of your genes, you are by no means out of danger.

The Western diet is loaded with elements which interfere with the essential fatty acid enzymes, like saturated fat and the chemically altered fats in margarine. These block the cellular production lines*, starving the body of the essential fatty acid derivatives it needs. In addition, many of the co-nutrients vital for these enzymes, such as zinc and magnesium, are in short supply because of food processing, and because commercial fertilizers don't replenish all the minerals taken from the soil by food crops. These fertilizers only supply nitrogen, phosphorus and potassium in abundance, supporting bountiful growth – but plants can get by with far fewer minerals than we can. This means that you could be suffering the effects of functional essential fatty acid deficiency *even if you follow government dietary recommendations and do not belong to a vulnerable racial group.*

## The Prostaglandin Factor

Medical journals are now starting to carry cautiously optimistic articles about essential fatty acids, especially since in 1985 fish oils were shown to reduce the risk of heart disease. But the cutting edge of research today concerns the *prostaglandins***, hormone-like substances made from essential fatty acids in every cell to regulate moment-to-moment conditions. Hormones differ from prostaglandins in that, while hormones are made in the

*These 'anti-nutrients' interfere with the enzymes which make prostaglandins, nerves and blood vessels from the EFAs.

**There are three families of prostaglandins, known as the PG1s, PG2s and PG3s. The 1s and 2s are derived from the *linoleic* acid in seed oils, while the 3s are made from *linolenic* acid derivatives found in seafood. In each family, different prostaglandins are classified with a letter of the alphabet – PGE1 and PGI2 are examples.

glands and act all over the body, prostaglandins can be made by every cell and act locally in the tissues where they were created.

In the arteries, for example, prostaglandins control how readily the blood will clot, muscular tension in the arterial wall (which affects blood pressure), and how easily a clot can attach itself to the arterial wall. Unlike hormones, prostaglandins' lives are necessarily very short, since their purpose is to help local tissues adapt quickly to changing conditions. This made them so elusive that, until recently, their widespread influence wasn't appreciated.

The same prostaglandin may also have several different functions. For example, prostaglandin E1 (PGE1) lessens clotting and dilates the blood vessels, and appears to lower cholesterol production in the liver.

Essential fatty acids have other functions in the body, notably in cell walls, where they control fluidity* and act as gatekeepers, helping control access to the cell. But prostaglandins seem to be the key to the incredible diversity of diseases in which functional deficiencies of the two essential fatty acids are involved.

## *Omega Oils*

The various fatty acids are classified by something called the 'omega notation', scientific shorthand for identifying the structure of an oil. The two fatty acids which are 'essential' belong to the omega-3 and omega-6 families. For our purposes, all we need remember is that omega-3 oils come from fish, omega-6 oils from plants.

As in every medical advance, the old guard has been slow to appreciate the importance of essential fatty acids and prostaglandins. Nutritional 'revolutionaries' such as Dr Donald Rudin (American researcher and author of *The Omega-3 Phenomenon***) claim there's so much to be gained with so little risk that new dietary recommendations should be made at once, before research finally dots the i's and crosses the t's.

The public evidently agrees with him, and so do I. Since fish

*Red blood cells must be flexible enough to fold almost in half to get through capillaries.

**Sidgwick and Jackson, London, 1988

oils have been publicized as being good for the heart, the sales of books with 'Omega' in their titles have grown, and there has been an upsurge in the demand for fish oil supplements. However, there is much more to this than just protection against heart disease, as we shall see.

## *Getting Started*

When Laura first asked if I knew of anything which might help her premenstrual tension (PMT), I asked if she had any other problems. Since she has blue eyes and blond hair, I thought that she might have a Scandinavian background. It turned out that she did. Her grandmother was born in Denmark. As the tell-tale complex of symptoms emerged – overweight, an allergy to wheat, irritability and depression – my suspicions were confirmed. Laura had strayed too far from her hereditary diet, and her body was rebelling.

I learned about my own hereditary diet problems first hand, whilst trying to work out a diet to help my diabetes. I tried the diabetic exchange diet, complex carbohydrates, macrobiotics and all the other supposed cure-alls I could find, but my food cravings and mood swings persisted, along with wild excursions of my blood sugar. Eventually, I did find that simple, unprocessed foods prepared with the least amount of cooking helped the most – but my problems were far from over.

I learned of research which showed that a *high-essential-fatty-acid-diet protects diabetics against the heart and blood vessel complications of diabetes*[9]. It seemed to me that because diabetes merely exaggerates the 'normal' incidence of cardiovascular disease, anything which helped diabetics would also be effective in people who did not have the disease. Then I came across an article in a medical journal about how diseases affect the prostaglandins, and I realized that the high blood sugar of diabetes lessens prostaglandin production, and that this effect must be responsible for many of the complications of diabetes. Ageing, genetic weakness and poor diet can do the same thing in normal people.

So I began eating foods like salmon and safflower oil which apparently promote production of the desirable prostaglandins while suppressing the undesirables, along with the vitamins and minerals which boost prostaglandin production. The difference was extraordinary. I had new energy, my weight began to fall, my mood settled several notches up from what I was used to and my blood-sugar control was better than ever before. My skin, hair and nails got stronger, and I felt years younger. I knew I had the answer, although it took me more than two years of experimentation to make it stick.

At long last, I was able to fulfil those 'eternal' New Year's resolutions to lose weight, eat a healthier diet and take life more calmly. This was the beginning of my formulation of a new way of eating, which I've called ***Food for Vitality.***

Laura might benefit from what I'd learned. Her prostaglandins were also disordered, although for a different reason. Her background meant a genetically weak essential fatty acid-to-prostaglandin pathway, and this frailty was being compounded by her diet. To get the ball rolling, I recommended that she should not eat wheat, since my own experience suggested that food-allergy problems don't resolve themselves unless the food is avoided.

Laura's food-allergy problem was that once she started eating bread, she couldn't stop. This craving so interfered with her appetite that she felt she couldn't control her weight, and her 'bread orgies' left her filled with self-disgust. Such food allergy/food addiction syndromes are thought to be caused by partially digested food fragments in the bloodstream* – more on this in Chapter 5, under 'Food Allergy, Food Addiction.'

Nick thought that avoiding bread sounded pretty restrictive, and that the 'hereditary diet' concept sounded highly unlikely. Exploring his background, I learned that Nick, who has classic Italian looks, was actually half Scottish. He told me about being tired in the evenings, his high risk factors for heart disease (overweight, high blood pressure and high cholesterol), and of regularly needing a drink to relax after work. It looked as if Nick's prostaglandins were also out of kilter.

*One theory has it that antigen-induced alterations to the immune-system 'complement cascade' cause the brain to regard the food much as it would a painkiller, although this is highly speculative. Whatever the explanation, however, the *observation* that some problems resolve themselves when over-used foods are removed from the diet has been made too often to be ignored.

I thought there was a good chance that his problems might respond to the same programme I was suggesting for Laura, except for avoiding bread. I proposed that they both try my prostaglandin-correcting ***Food for Vitality*** eating plan, which is outlined below and explained in detail in the next chapter. They agreed to suspend their disbelief and undertake the programme for a trial period.

Three months later, the change in Nick and Laura was extraordinary. They both looked less tired. The kids said that they nagged them less. Nick's energy was up and his wine consumption down. Feeling better meant he had less need for alcohol. The marks on his belt bore out his claim that he'd lost more than a few pounds. Afternoons at the office were no longer a battle against sleepiness, and his furies and indigestion rarely bothered him any more. A recent checkup revealed a decrease of both blood pressure and cholesterol.

Laura was much less irritable with the children, although if anything her allergies seemed worse. When I asked in what way, she laughed, sheepishly admitting to trying bread every so often 'just to see if my craving's still there!'* Her nails were definitely stronger, however. But the big news concerned her premenstrual tension. After little change during the first month, her symptoms were less severe by the second and vastly improved by the third!

What thrilled her most was her increased ability to handle pressure and stress without losing composure. I was sure that this was the result of a strengthened essential fatty acid-to-prostaglandin pathway being better able to withstand the inhibiting effect of the stress hormone adrenalin. A strong pathway can shrug off the effects of a lot more adrenalin and still produce mood-enhancing prostaglandin E1 (PGE1). In other words, *your ability to handle stress may depend more on your diet than the amount of stress you're under.*

Since PGE1 improves mood, one's less likely to become irritated

*If a person is allergic to one food, they're usually allergic to several. Food allergies improve very slowly on the ***Food for Vitality*** programme unless the problem food is avoided completely – the immune system has a long memory. However, while a 'healthy' appetite can become a positive craving for the food when it is first avoided, this excess appetite just melts away after a few days.

by stressful circumstances. Therefore, as with hostility and heart attacks, it seems likely that *stress* and *distress* may actually be two effects linked by low prostaglandins, rather than being cause and effect.

Initially, Nick and Laura had felt trapped. That had been my feeling, too – that I was locked into an endless cycle of not feeling well and not knowing why. The sense of relief experienced by all three of us, resulting from the realization that there *is* something we can do that is manageable, has been profound.

Now it's your turn. Together, let's take a look at the diet which has made such a difference to Nick and Laura's lives – a diet which can do the same for you. We'll begin with the next chapter, in which I describe the ***Food for Vitality*** programme in detail.

# 2: What to Eat to Feel Terrific

***The food question is infinitely the most important problem of the present day – and if properly dealt with must result in the disappearance of the vast bulk of disease, misery and death.***

SIR WILLIAM ARBUTHNOT LANE, MD (*1846–1943*)

The ***Food for Vitality*** plan is the cornerstone of this book, the result of my efforts to discover a way of eating which corrects disordered essential fatty acid metabolism and alleviates the various ailments we've been discussing. Many people have tried it, and it's helped young and old alike.

This is not a rigid menu plan advocating 8 apricots on Monday, 3 ounces of tuna on Tuesday and so forth. Rather, these are recommendations for a *new pattern of eating*, an overall approach which allows you flexibility in your daily eating choices.

Laura told me that even though she and Nick had managed to follow the plan only about 60% of the time, they'd both improved tremendously. This brings out another important point: THIS IS NOT AN ALL-OR-NOTHING DIET. It will still be effective if you simply eat this way more often than not. It's entirely human to break diets, and the important thing is to forgive yourself and go back on the plan. If you must down three bottles of champagne to celebrate Granny's 100th birthday – enjoy them! But start the ***Food for Vitality*** programme again at breakfast.

The encouraging thing about the ***Food for Vitality*** programme is that the longer you stay on it, the easier it is to follow, because this way of eating seems to lessen the cravings which make other diets so difficult to maintain.

The basic elements of my ***Food for Vitality*** programme are summarized below. Read them through, and don't worry if some of them don't make much sense to you right now. They will, because in this chapter I'll be taking the points in turn, explaining fully and clearly the scientific reasons behind them, and how you can work them into your daily life with a minimum of fuss.

At the end of this section, I've given a typical sample day of food suggestions to show you how it works in practice.

## *Food For Vitality*

1. Eat fish instead of meat, and take evening primrose oil (to assure sufficient essential fatty acid derivatives)*.
2. Use cold-pressed, unrefined flaxseed (linseed) and safflower oil for salad dressings, olive oil for cooking.
3. Cut down on saturated fat (in red meat, baked goods and fried foods) and hydrogenated oils (in margarine and refined vegetable oils).
4. Have no more than one egg and one glass of milk a day**.
5. Whenever possible, buy organic vegetables and fruit. In any case, as much as possible, eat vegetables and fruit uncooked.
6. Cut down on sugar, refined flour, alcohol and caffeine***.
7. Take supplements of *Optivite* (to boost the prostaglandin metabolism), and take vitamin C (to protect the delicate

*Evening primrose oil supplements are unnecessary if you're in perfect health. However, they are desirable if you should lean towards any of the conditions summarized in Chapter 5 (page 113), including ageing. Evening primrose oil's few side-effects are listed on pages 50-51.

**Assuming that you don't have adverse reactions to eggs or milk, and neither crave nor over-use them. Note that about 40% or more of the sub-population who 'feel poorly' have adverse reactions to milk! See 'Food Allergy, Food Addiction', page 151. See also Theron Randolph and Ralph Moss, *An Alternative Approach to Allergies*, Harper and Row, New York, 1980.

***Any whose cravings are such that they cannot cut down should eliminate the offending food. Although this may sound harsh, my experience has been that severe food allergies can sabotage the benefits of this programme. *Avoid the foods you can't control.*

essential fatty acids and the cholesterol in your bloodstream – see page 170.

8. Take soluble fibre supplements if you don't enjoy consummate regularity.

To see how these guidelines actually translate into food, glance through the following menu suggestions. As you can see from the food choices, a prostaglandin-supporting diet can be delicious – in fact, it's absolutely vital that the food should be delicious because nobody can continue to eat an unpalatable diet, however convinced of its healthful effects they may be.

## FOOD FOR A DAY

### CHOOSE ONE SELECTION AT EACH MEAL

### BREAKFAST

1. Half a grapefruit or an orange, followed by a boiled free-range egg with wholemeal toast soldiers 'buttered' with flaxseed (linseed) oil. To save time, I buy lots of stone-ground wholemeal bread and freeze it until needed.
2. Porridge, served with a little low-fat milk or yoghurt. A dollop of apple sauce makes a delicious sweetener.
3. Muesli, soaked overnight in low-fat milk and topped with chopped apple. Be sure to choose a sugar-free variety of packaged muesli. If you like, add some soaked sunflower seeds (rich in omega-6 oils) and walnuts (for the omega-3s).

### *Supplements*

Take three or four *Efamol* evening primrose oil capsules and two *Optivite.* You can also take your fibre supplement at breakfast, either mixed in fruit juice or stirred into muesli or porridge.

### *What to Drink*

You can drink decaffeinated tea or coffee*, herb teas or coffee substitutes anytime, all through the day. Keep supplies at the office

*Decaffeinated coffee contains theobromine and other potential villains whose inflammatory effects in the gut may exacerbate food allergies. If in doubt, avoid.

– or carry your own tea bags in your briefcase or handbag for restaurants which don't serve decaffeinated drinks. Fruit juices drunk on their own contain so much readily-available sugar that they suppress the immune system[1], so it's always better to eat the whole fruit. Taking your fibre supplement in fruit juice is all right, however, because the fibre slows sugar absorption.

## ELEVENSES

1. Mixed nuts and raisins. A good combination is walnuts, sunflower seeds and raisins, with Grape Nuts if you like extra crunch.

2. Home-made nutty oatmeal biscuits – delicious straight from the oven, or can be frozen until needed.

3. An apple with a handful of walnuts (walnuts contain some omega-3 oil).

## LUNCH

### *1. Restaurants:*

**Indian**: tandoori chicken, curried vegetables, cucumber raita and nan (a bread).
**International or eclectic**: poached salmon, try for double raw vegetables and go easy on the white rolls and butter.
**Thai**: prawns with ginger and vegetables.
**Italian**: I like to start with the biggest salad on the menu, followed by pasta shells with pesto sauce, but stay away from creamy dishes like Fettucine Alfredo and cannelloni.
**French**: Sauces loaded with delicious but deadly fat are the big problem here – go for the fish grilled with lemon juice (sauce on the side) and a big salad.

### *2. At home:*

Try a salad Niçoise, or sardines and CRUNCHY SALAD (a perennial standby made of whatever's in season, such as organically grown carrots, red and green peppers, cucumber, peas, spinach, Jerusalem artichokes, etc. Make enough for two days and store in the fridge). Or a Greek Salad of tomatoes, cucumber, onions, Provençale olives and a little feta cheese with bread drizzled with a mixture of virgin olive and flaxseed (linseed) oils.

### 3. *Take-to-the-office/school lunch:*

Chicken or tuna and watercress sandwiches on wholewheat bread with carrot sticks. Or brown pita-pockets filled with CRUNCHY SALAD dressed with guacamole and a thermos of home-made SPLIT-PEA SOUP.

## Dinner

### 1. *In a hurry?*

Serve an appetizer of raw corn-on-the-cob (organically grown corn usually tastes better, and it must be fresh as you can get it), brushed with just enough flaxseed (linseed) oil to get freshly ground pepper and sea-salt to stick. Follow with an omelette aux fines herbes or scrambled eggs with smoked salmon (save up your egg allowance for these), with previously made CRUNCHY SALAD.

### 2. *Entertaining dinner guests?*

Start with half an avocado filled with prawns and flaxseed (linseed)/olive oil vinaigrette, then serve grilled trout stuffed with mint and stir-fried vegetables with a little brown rice. Blackberries with a low-fat yoghurt make a refreshing dessert.

### 3. *At home for the evening?*

Serve GAZPACHO soup, made in the food processor from tomatoes, cucumbers, peppers, oil, garlic and onion. Follow with a baked potato filled with low-fat yoghurt and chives or HOME-BAKED BEANS, accompanied by a walnut, basil and tomato salad. Alternatively, serve scallops stir-fried with herbs and garlic, with a CRUNCHY SALAD – which you can also stir-fry, if you like. Or try my favourite VEGETABLE TOSTADA – bake corn tortillas (find them in an international delicatessen) until crisp in a hot oven, spread with avocado and cover with CRUNCHY SALAD. Top with a dressing of olive oil, flaxseed (linseed) oil, lemon juice, garlic, salt and pepper, with anchovies *or* feta cheese for flavour, all whizzed up in the food processor. Garnish with sliced boiled baby beets and serve with stir-fried salmon.

*Supplements*

Repeat as at breakfast.

If this kind of eating pattern supplies most of your calories, you can easily weather the occasional chocolate biscuit attack or dinner at your mother's.

Now let's examine the ***Food for Vitality*** suggestions one at a time, from the top.

## 1. Eat Fish Instead Of Meat, And Take Evening Primrose Oil

### Eat Fish Instead of Meat

Putting this into action is as easy as choosing poached salmon instead of pork chops when eating out, making a chef's salad with sardines instead of cheese at home, or taking a tuna sandwich instead of ham to the office for lunch. The reason for it is simple. The important thing about these food choices is that they all supply omega-3 essential fatty acids*.

I suspect that the most pervasive diet problem today is a lack of such oils, which are found in cold-water fish**. Unlike wild game, domestic livestock have almost none, except in the parts we don't eat. And omega-3 oils are *intentionally* destroyed in refined oils and margarines in order to prevent rancidity, while milling removes them from grains with the bran. As a result, only about one fifth of what was in the diet at the turn of the century remains in the food available today, and this may be too little to sustain health.

This doesn't mean you've got to eat fish at every meal – chicken

*For example, eicosapentanoic acid (EPA) and docosahexanoic acid (DHA) are in the news often these days.

**Not only the amounts of, but also the *ratio* between the essential fatty acids is wrong in our diet. We eat between 10 and 14 times more of the omega-6, land-based fatty acids than of the omega-3, ocean-based family, whereas the ideal ratio is thought to lie between 1:1 and 6:1 (A. Simopoulos, 'w-3 Fatty Acids in Growth . . . and in Health and Disease', *Nutrition Today*, May/June 1988).

is an alternative. Although it has little in the way of essential fatty acids, chicken contains much less of the harmful saturated fat found in red meat*. Steak eaten occasionally isn't going to kill you – although it very well might if you were to eat it every day.

As few as three fish meals a week will make a big difference, although more is even better. Heart attack risk is actually halved when an average of just one ounce of fish is eaten daily – which also means that the omega-3 oils are powerful stuff indeed, and that most people apparently need them badly!

The retina of the eye is very rich in omega-3 oils, and the fats in the brain are about half and half omega-3 and omega-6, which shows just how highly the body values the omega-3s since they're so scarce in the diet. In addition to forming some of our most valuable tissues, omega-3 oils also help regulate the prostaglandins.

Fish-eaters tend to have more desirable 1- and 3-series prostaglandins in their tissues. Those who lean towards meat, eggs and milk may have more of the 2-series prostaglandins which prepare the body for stressful conditions by making the blood more likely to clot and by constricting the blood vessels. In fact, the 'eicosapentanoic acid' or EPA found in fish is a more effective blood thinner than aspirin, alcohol or even streptokinase, the miracle 'clot-busting' enzyme given to heart attack victims. Consequently, high blood pressure and heart attacks are much more common on meat diets, while fish protects against them.

This arrangement (the type of prostaglandin which gets made depending on what is eaten) looks like Nature's mistake until you consider that our diets were very different during the evolution of the human race. What little fat there was on the wild game eaten by early hunters was mostly essential, whereas the meat we eat today is loaded with saturated fat which clogs up the whole essential fatty acid system. Similarly, wild plants contain far more omega-3s than cultivated varieties. So we tried to fool Nature

*A wild pheasant is about 3% fat by weight, and a chicken carcass was about 2.4% fat in 1900. However, modern broiler-house techniques have upped chickens to 22%! The equivalent figures for wild buffalo and domestic cattle are about 2% and 25%, respectively.

with our modern diet and clever farming methods, but Nature has the last laugh since we've saddled ourselves with a tendency towards high blood pressure and heart attacks.

*The reason men are more prone to heart attacks is probably because they have two to three times the essential fatty acid requirement of women*[2]. During pregnancy, females become tremendously depleted of essential fatty acids from building the baby's brain and nervous system, so their bodies have adapted to get by on less for periods of time. But this protection disappears after the child-bearing years, when women's heart attack risk rises rapidly towards that of men.

I suspect the profound depression some mothers go through after giving birth – post-partum depression (or even psychosis) – may also be caused by this depletion, which could reduce desirable prostaglandin E1 to the levels thought to exist in people with severe depression*.

Omega-3 oils are made by plankton in cold waters because such heavily polyunsaturated oils stay liquid at low temperatures, and work like anti-freeze – the colder the water, the more omega-3 oils the plankton make. In the ocean, krill (tiny shrimp) acquire the oils when they eat the plankton, and so on up the food chain. Thus, cold-water ocean fish like salmon, as well as some fresh-water fish like rainbow trout (if they're from cold waters such as in Lake Superior), contain plentiful EPA. Fish are almost the only 'wild game' still available to us.

Land sources of omega-3s include flaxseed (linseed), pumpkin seeds, walnuts and green leafy vegetables, and, as with fish, the cold-adapted, northerly varieties contain the most omega-3.

*Prostaglandins must be hedged about with 'mays', 'coulds' and 'thought to be's' because their lives are so fleeting that it's almost impossible to measure levels in living tissue. The interference caused by the measuring equipment alone can raise some prostaglandin levels by some *ten thousand* times! Researchers must therefore concentrate on fatty acid levels, or deduce prostaglandin levels from some other observation. Hence, the low prostaglandin E1 'levels thought to exist in people with severe depression' are inferred from the lessened ability of depressives' platelets to make prostaglandin E1 when stimulated in the laboratory (Y. Abdullah et al., 'Effect of ADP on PGE Formation in Blood Platelets from Patients with Depression, Mania and Schizophrenia', *British Journal of Psychiatry*, 1975, 127:591-595).

## WHAT KIND OF FISH?

When choosing your fish from the menu or fish shop, here's what to bear in mind*. The fish richest in omega-3 oils are salmon, sardines, albacore tuna and mackerel – all have dark-coloured flesh. Herring, swordfish, bass, red snapper, Atlantic halibut and yellowfin tuna contain middling amounts. So do scallops, prawns and other shellfish, although those from colder waters such as the North Sea will contain more than those from southerly waters. Carp, perch, Pacific halibut, haddock, cod, pike and sole are low in omega-3 oils (although cod have plenty in their oily livers). Farmed fish have little omega-3 unless their feed contained these oils, which is unlikely** – although chickens have been fed omega-3 oils to lower the cholesterol content of their eggs.

Unfortunately, a trip to the local fish-and-chip shop is not going to do the trick – fish-fingers, fried fish and fast-food 'fish-wiches' won't have much protective effect. They're usually made from fish poor in essential fatty acids, and come wrapped in crunchy coatings which contain many times as much oil as the fish itself, but of the wrong kind.

## TAKE EVENING PRIMROSE OIL

Another way to help your body make the right prostaglandins is to take evening primrose oil capsules. The seeds of the evening primrose are most unusual because they contain pre-formed gamma-linolenic acid, or GLA, which is what the body tries to make from essential omega-6 oils in food.

One reason that GLA is important is because prostaglandin E1 (PGE1) can be made from it. PGE1 is a wonderfully useful

*Pollution worries many people, and one estimate of the increased risk of eating trout from Lake Ontario weekly is 1 in 200 – about the same risk as being murdered if you live in the United States! Trout fishing is now banned in this heavily polluted lake, but pollution can reach similar levels offshore from major cities. Tips for avoiding pollution from a US consumer newsletter include eating a wide variety, avoiding fish caught in coastal waters, eating small fish which haven't had time to accumulate much pollution, minimizing raw fish consumption and avoiding the 'mustard' (liver and pancreas) in lobsters because of cadmium and PCB accumulation (*Nutrition Action Healthletter*, October 1988).

**Some fish-farm feeds are reputed to contain sewage sludge!

prostaglandin which boosts the immune system, lowers cholesterol and blood pressure and apparently also improves the mood! GLA also kills cancer cells in the laboratory and has reduced tumour size in laboratory animals, which suggests that functional essential fatty acid deficiencies have a lot to do with our extraordinarily high rate of cancer.

## ALCOHOL

Prostaglandin E1 (PGE1) has profound effects on how we feel. It's thought to be almost undetectable in schizophrenics, low in depressives and chronic alcoholics, and very high in the euphoric, 'up' phase of manic depression. One reason Nick's evening drinks made him feel better is that alcohol stimulates PGE1 production, which improves mood. However, alcohol also slows production of PGE1's precursors. This means less PGE1 when the alcohol wears off, and no doubt accounts for the truth of the saying:

***A drink makes me feel like a new man. Unfortunately, the first thing the new man wants is another drink.***

ANON

Since evening primrose by-passes this first step and supplies GLA ready-made, it raises PGE1 – and this, marvellous to relate, is said to actually reduce the desire for alcohol! In fact, I've seen this programme lessen consumption in social drinkers, without major efforts of will on their part*.

When research studies showed that alcohol protects against heart attacks, both the drink manufacturers and heavy drinkers alike grabbed hold of this tidbit like drowning sailors. However, the protective effect of alcohol is quite small, and disappears if more or less than two drinks per day are taken**.

Since alcohol stimulates PGE1 production while at the same

*However, alcoholics may actually drink more on evening primrose oil.

**It may not even be the alcohol that has the protective effect. Beer drinking rats had considerably more copper in their livers than rats given alcohol and water to drink, even though the beer contained only traces of copper. Something in the beer apparently enhanced the rats' ability to absorb copper from their diet, and it is well accepted that copper deficiency raises cholesterol levels ('Give that Rat a Bud', *Discover*, September, 1990).

time lessening the capacity to make PGE1 in the future, two drinks a day may be just the right amount for a little extra protective PGE1 at the expense of depleting the DGLA stored in cell membranes. This could only work if PGE1 were chronically low – as it probably is in the meat-eating American population in which it was found. This implies, however, that normal everyday PGE1 levels must decline in time because alcohol interferes with the all-important initial step in which dietary linoleic acid is converted into PGE1's precursors. In this model of alcoholism, the lowered PGE1 triggers an increased desire for alcohol.

My experience confirms this – people have either little interest or far too much interest in alcohol, and those who continue to drink two drinks a day are very few and far between. Increasing PGE1 production with fish and evening primrose oil is a better strategy than just consuming alcohol, because it improves the mood naturally and protects the heart more effectively than alcohol, without alcohol's debilitating effects. This strategy also makes drinking much easier to control and tends to lessen consumption, a boon for those who have trouble controlling their alcohol intake.

## A More Direct Route

The body can make its own GLA (the active substance in evening primrose oil) from the essential omega-6 linoleic acid, or LA, found in green leafy vegetables and vegetable oils, sunflower seeds, wheat germ, walnuts and pumpkin seeds. But since the conversion of LA to GLA can be blocked by genetic weakness, ageing, viral infections or poor diet, it makes sense to by-pass this step by supplying the body with GLA ready-made in evening primrose oil.

## The Cholesterol Factor

The GLA in evening primrose oil lowers cholesterol 170–700% more effectively than the LA in vegetable oil from which GLA is made in the body, so a working essential fatty acid pathway appears crucial for a normal cholesterol level[3]. In one experiment, evening primrose oil lowered starting cholesterol levels of 7* or more to an average of 5.3 – a reduction of 24%. The higher the initial cholesterol level, the greater the lowering effect[4].

This incredible (and virtually unpublicized) result renders cholesterol-lowering drugs like cholestyramine, lovastatin and clofibrate, with all their dangerous side-effects, obsolete. *The GLA in evening primrose oil is the most potent cholesterol-lowering agent on the face of the earth!*

## What to Take

There are many brands of evening primrose oil available in chemists and health food shops**. *Efamol* is a well-known and reliable brand which has been shown in clinical trials to help all sorts of problems linked to low PGE1, such as PMT, irritability, high cholesterol and poor skin. Dr David Horrobin (an English-born doctor who researches in Canada) instigated most of the *Efamol* research, and has been scrupulous in ensuring that the studies are scientifically respectable. When I buy it, I console myself that some of its high price goes to fund further research.

Six capsules of *Efamol* contain 270 mg of GLA, about twice the GLA a baby gets – but only if it's breast-fed, since cow's milk has almost none***.

## How the Body Forms Prostaglandins

A diagram of the essential fatty acid-to-prostaglandin pathway is shown opposite to help make clear what we're trying to do, which is to boost 1-prostaglandin production.

From the diagram, you can see that evening primrose oil boosts GLA, by-passing the 'delicate first step' in which GLA is made

*Units are millimoles per litre.

**Borage seed, blackcurrant seed and even fungus oil contains GLA, but the only study ever performed on their relative merits indicated that evening primrose oil is by far the most effective source. See page 101 for more on this.

***The evening primrose oil should supply between 4 and 10 times as much omega-6 GLA as the sum of the omega-3 EPA and DHA from fish in the diet to maximize desirable prostaglandins while at the same time suppressing the trouble makers.

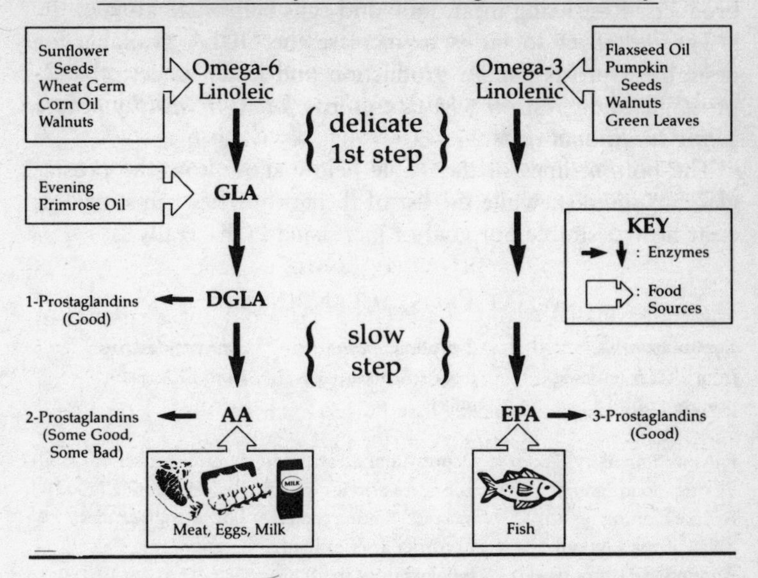


*Figure 1 The Essential Fatty Acid-to-Prostaglandin Pathway*

***The metabolic pathways of the essential fatty acids are well known, and since we can neither manufacture them nor convert one into the other, both are vital for good health. Only a tiny fraction of the EFAs we consume are made into prostaglandins, the messenger molecules which control local conditions all over the body, but without them there would be biological chaos. The PG1s and PG3s are 'good' because they promote healing, lower blood pressure and inhibit the PG2s. The PG2s are 'bad' because their 'prepare for fight or flight' message is usually a false alarm caused by the deficiencies of our Western diet.***

from the linoleic acid (LA) dietary vegetable oils*. Fish and fish oils increase EPA and encourage beneficial 3-prostaglandins which, with 1-prostaglandins, curb production of the undesirable

*Rates of conversion from LA to GLA in healthy tissues were found to be: Adrenals 20%, Liver 14%, Testes 6%, Heart, Kidney and Brain 1-2%. Most essential fatty acid conversion appears to take place in the liver.

2-prostaglandins made from the arachidonic acid (AA) in animal products. Restricting meat, milk and eggs helps here also.

The net effect so far is to increase the DGLA available for desirable 1-prostaglandin production and lessen undesirable 2-prostaglandins, *restoring levels to those found in healthy people eating traditional diets.*

The bottom lines of the Table below show how the prostaglandins interact, while the list of their properties helps make it clear how desirable our goal of increasing PGE1 really is.

## WHAT PROSTAGLANDINS DO

| *1-prostaglandins* from DGLA (evening primrose oil): | *2-prostaglandins* from AA (meat, eggs, milk): | *3-prostaglandins* from EPA (fish): |
|---|---|---|
| Enhance immunity (good) | Depress immunity (bad) | Lubricate arteries (good) |
| Elevate mood (good) | Lubricate arteries (good) | Reduce clotting (good) |
| Reduce clotting (good) | Increase clotting (bad) | Lower triglycerides (good) |
| Relax arteries (good) | Constrict arteries (bad) | |
| Anti-inflammatory (good) | Inflammatory (bad) | |
| Lower cholesterol (good) | | |
| Activate brown fat (good) | | |
| Inhibit 2-prostaglandins by slowing AA release | Inhibit 1-prostaglandin production from DGLA | Inhibit 2-prostaglandins by slowing AA production |

Thus, the combination of fish and evening primrose oil bypasses the 'delicate first step' in the essential fatty acid-to- prostaglandin pathway, and also encourages desirable 1-prostaglandin production. However, *too much* EPA* can inhibit the 1-prostaglandins as well as the 2-prostaglandins – which could be why the leading cause of death among Eskimos is infection, since 1-prostaglandins boost immunity. This is one of many good reasons *not* to take vast quantities of fish oil.

*EPA itself produces some of these effects. For example, giving huge amounts of fish oil practically closes down the prostaglandin metabolism by crowding out other essential fatty acids, and still lowers triglycerides.

The 'delicate first step' in the diagram is weak in some people for genetic reasons, and declines in all of us with age. This step is easily blocked by a number of factors, including the stress-hormone adrenalin, saturated fat (in meat, baked goods and fried foods), cholesterol, sugar, alcohol and the hydrogenates in margarine, baked goods and refined vegetable oils.

- Foods rich in saturated fat like whole milk
- Foods rich in cholesterol like red meat
- The stress hormones adrenaline and cortisol
- Low levels of zinc, magnesium, vitamins B6 or B3, which are common in the UK because of food refining
- Alcohol in excess of two glasses of wine per day or the equivalent
- Allergies and other atopic conditions like eczema
- High blood sugar, as in diabetes
- Ageing
- Viral infections
- Cancer

It's important to realize that until dietary essential fatty acids pass this 'delicate first step', *they have little essential activity in the body* (other than maintaining skin and cell wall structure) and are mostly used for calories. This is why preserving elements of the hereditary diet which promote prostaglandin production is vitally important for people such as the aged, the genetically vulnerable and those under stress, and why the pattern of eating described here is so very effective for almost everybody.

Although prostaglandin effects are newly discovered, we're actually not strangers to them. For example, most of aspirin's effects exist because aspirin inhibits enzymes which make prostaglandins from the essential fatty acids. Interestingly, large doses of vitamin C control inflammation, fever and pain by inhibiting undesirable prostaglandins, but such doses actually *encourage* beneficial prostaglandin E1 production[5].

There is even a controversial method for reducing heart attacks which relies on aspirin's prostaglandin-inhibiting effect. This strategy halved heart attacks in a group of American doctors who acted as guinea pigs in a study, and cut heart attacks in British doctors by a third*. It probably works, when it works, by destroying the enzymes in blood platelets which make artery-choking 2-prostaglandins, but leaving the same enzymes intact in the cells lining the arteries, where they make protective, clot-busting prostacyclin. Aspirin's protective effect disappears when it's taken every day (as in rheumatoid arthritis), since this destroys the enzymes in the cells lining the arteries as well as in the platelets.

Compare this crude approach with the ***Food for Vitality*** programme, which harnesses the full potential of the protective prostaglandins while inhibiting the destructive varieties. And it seems likely that by compensating for our declining essential fatty acid pathway, the ***Food for Vitality*** programme can literally reverse a second familiar group of prostaglandin-directed effects, the changes of ageing. But before we get into that, what about evening primrose oil's side effects?

## Evening Primrose Oil's Side Effects?

Almost anything can be detrimental if it's taken in too high a dose, but evening primrose oil's side-effects are remarkably benign. Evening primrose oil's sebum-thinning effect which so helped my blackheads sometimes causes hard cysts under the skin in those prone to such cysts. Theory suggests that starting to eat lots of fish some time before commencing the evening primrose oil will prevent this.

I've found the early-morning insomnia which too much evening primrose oil can cause to be more of a blessing than a drawback, since I've always been dopey in the mornings. Lessening the dose is the remedy for those who want to sleep in. A temporary euphoria seems to be a related side effect, although I thoroughly enjoyed it for the four days it lasted when I first took evening primrose oil.

*The difference may be because the US doctors took 325 mg every other day (*New England Journal of Medicine*, 28 January 1988), while the UK doctors took 500 mg (*British Medical Journal*, 30 January 1988). Some believe the higher levels in the British study cut protective prostacyclin in production in the blood vessel walls. Interestingly, the aspirin also cut migraines by 20% in the American doctors (*Science News*, 1990, 137(7):102).

Temporal-lobe epilepsy may be confused with schizophrenia, but while evening primrose oil reportedly improves those aspects of schizophrenia which do not respond to drugs, temporal lobe epilepsy is worsened. People prone to migraines have reported more frequent attacks on evening primrose oil. Usually these are the same people for whom alcohol triggers migraines, and Cytotec* is protective for some. Finally, increased menstrual flow, increased bleeding time (from cuts, etc.), minor headaches, nausea and a low incidence of diarrhoea have also been reported[6].

It is encouraging that in Canada and Sweden, with more than 100 million *Efamol* capsules consumed in each country per annum, not a single complaint had been received by the licensing authorities[7].

## LOOK YOUNGER LONGER

With advancing age, cholesterol levels and heart disease rise steeply. Skin loses its youthful glow and becomes lifeless and wrinkled, and many people become more irritable and short-tempered. Two problems with the immune system become more prevalent. First, declining activity of the cells which damp down the immune response allows increased auto-immune disease (such as rheumatoid arthritis and multiple sclerosis), in which the body's immune system mistakenly attacks parts of the body itself. Second, a progressive failure of 'immune surveillance' permits more cancer**.

It is entirely possible that all this deterioration stems from the age-related decline in our ability to convert LA into GLA in the 'delicate first step' of the essential fatty acid-to-prostaglandin pathway. Without sufficient GLA, we can't make enough soothing 1-prostaglandins. But, at the same time, a diet rich in meat, eggs and milk supplies plentiful AA, so the pathway machinery works unrestrained to create inflammatory, immune-system-

*A long-acting analogue of prostaglandin E1 made by Searle Laboratories – see page 153.

**The second effect may stem from the first. If the immune system is worn out from attacking everything in sight, its effectiveness against real threats must be diminished.

suppressing 2-prostaglandins. These may cause problems such as arthritis, for which we take aspirin – but aspirin in quantity cancels our remaining capacity for making the 1-prostaglandins. *This must inevitably cause further deterioration* eventually because it's the 1-prostaglandins which promote healing and tissue repair.*

Interestingly, people with diabetes and rheumatoid arthritis are notoriously bad at staying on their therapeutic diets, as indicated by articles in the medical literature with titles like 'Diet Therapy for Diabetes: An Analysis of Failure.'[8] Since the essential fatty acids may have to do with food cravings and are low in both diseases, perhaps sufferers' excessive appetites will eventually be discovered to be related to their diseases, rather than blamed on their lack of will-power. The ***Food for Vitality*** approach seems to return the power of choice to both diabetics and rheumatoid arthritics.

## 2. Use Cold-Pressed, Unrefined Flaxseed and Safflower Oil for Salad Dressings, Olive Oil For Cooking

### Use Cold-Pressed, Unrefined Flaxseed and Safflower Oil for Salad Dressings

We're all well aware of the thousand and one bottled salad dressings available in the supermarket. Unfortunately, all of them contain oils which are bad for you. However, cold-pressed, unrefined safflower oil is rich in linoleic acid, the omega-6 essential fatty acid, while flaxseed oil is rich in both omega-3 and omega-6 essential fatty acids. Nutritionally speaking, either flaxseed or safflower oil is an improvement on olive oil, which contains almost no essential fatty acids. However, there's no

*Evidence for this comes from a 1989 University of Southern California Medical School study headed by Dr Annlia Paganni-Hill which found that taking an aspirin a day dramatically increased the risk of colon and kidney cancer among 14,000 retired persons.

denying that olive oil tastes great – so the ideal salad oil may well be equal parts of olive, flaxseed (linseed)* and safflower oils.

To save the bother of making a salad dressing at each meal, I make up a batch which will last about a week and keep it in the fridge. I always choose the darkest, murkiest oil with the most sediment for salad dressings, because although refining may create an attractive-looking, light-tasting oil, some of the linoleic acid will be damaged and no longer useful as essential fatty acid. Also, the protective natural antioxidant vitamin E remains intact in such oils.

Look for flaxseed oil in health food shops. It is also called food grade linseed oil – not to be confused with paint-base** or the stuff you put on cricket bats! – and has long been consumed in Germany, where it's considered part of a prudent diet.

Flaxseed oil is unusual among vegetable oils because it contains plentiful omega-3 linolenic acid, or LNA, from which the essential fatty acid pathway enzymes (if they're in working order) can make EPA (see page 47). However, the essential fatty acids in flaxseed oil are very delicate, so the flax seeds must be cold-pressed (below 40°C), and the oil cannot be refined or deodorized – it must even be protected from light and oxygen, which cause rancidity. Bioceuticals is a British manufacturer who packages flaxseed oil properly protected under nitrogen in opaque plastic containers***.

LNA only joined the essential fatty acids in 1982, when a six-year-old girl who was being fed intravenously because of a gunshot wound developed difficulty walking and numb patches on her legs. Changing her formula to include more LNA cured these symptoms, and her doctors concluded that LNA is indeed essential for humans.

*Flaxseed oil contains 50% linolenic acid and 22% linoleic acid, so it is an incredibly rich source of the omega-3 essential fatty acid.

**Flaxseed (linseed) and safflower oil contain very few antioxidants, which is why a solid skin forms on an open can of (linseed) oil-base paint – the oxygen of the air reacts with and 'cross-links' the unprotected oil. A similar reaction takes place in the body if there are too few antioxidants, contributing to wrinkled skin, liver spots etc.

***Bioceuticals Limited (Linseed Oil), 26 Zennor Road, London SW12 0PS, Tel. 081 675-5664.

## Use Olive Oil for Cooking

Since flaxseed and safflower oil contain so much delicate essential fatty acid, they smoke at quite low temperatures and aren't useful for cooking*. Olive oil, however, is stable when heated. It has another benefit – Mediterranean populations who eat it have fewer heart attacks than we do. This is probably because olives give up their oil easily and the harsh, fatty-acid-damaging extraction methods needed to get oil out of crops like maize aren't necessary, and the fatty acids in olive oil remain undamaged. Damaged fatty acids interfere with the essential fatty acid-to-prostaglandin pathway, increasing heart attack risk, so even though olive oil contains few essential fatty acids, it is the better choice for cooking.

# 3. Cut Down on Saturated Fat and Hydrogenated Oils

## Cut Down on Saturated Fat

By now, most people have heard quite a bit about the health dangers of those villainous saturated fats found in meat, fried foods, dairy products, etc. Some believe that saturated fats clog the prostaglandin machinery, lessening 1-prostaglandin production and so contributing to high cholesterol. If there's plentiful AA (from meat, eggs and milk) in the diet, then this may cause excess clot-promoting 2-prostaglandins to be produced. Consequently, meals rich in saturated fat give rise to blocked capillaries, simultaneously starving, asphyxiating and poisoning our most delicate tissues with their own waste!**

The major dietary sources of saturated fat are red meat and

*Oils which contain the EFAs are delicate! Their shelf lives are only a few months long, even when refrigerated in tightly-capped containers. Once opened, use them within six weeks to avoid rancidity.

**When coronary-prone men were given cream to drink, researchers could actually see delicate capillaries becoming blocked on the surface of their eyeballs! M. Friedman et al., 'Serum Lipids and Conjunctival Circulation after Fat Ingestion in Men Exhibiting Type-A Behaviour Pattern', Circulation Association, 1964, 29:874-886

whole milk, with frying fat and butter not far behind. Saturated vegetable fats include coconut and palm kernel oils (found in coffee whitener, biscuits and carob 'chocolate', among other foods), which are well-known to cause plaque, the porridge-like mass which forms on the lining of the arteries in heart disease. Unfortunately, products containing these oils are often misleadingly advertised as containing 'no cholesterol', despite the unquestionable fact that they're health-destroyers.

Butter and olive oil are stable when heated, and are therefore much healthier to cook with than delicate polyunsaturates, although olive oil is more desirable because it's *monounsaturated*, while butter is mostly saturated fat. Both are infinitely preferable to oils and margarines which have been refined or *hydrogenated.*

## Avoid Hydrogenates like the Plague!

Do you think that margarine is better for you than butter? Wrong! It's just another example of misleading advertising. In fact, the process of commercial oil and margarine production reads like an object lesson in how to destroy essential fatty acids. As crops like maize do not give up their oil without a struggle, damaging high temperatures and chemical solvents are used to help extraction. Further high-temperature processes (clarification, degumming, deodorizing) are then needed to make the light, clear oils we're used to.

Clarification of oils strips away the natural antioxidant vitamin E (which causes cloudiness), leaving a clear oil no longer protected against oxidation and rancidity. Its short shelf life would lead to commercial disaster but for hydrogenation, invented to take care of this problem.

Hydrogenation forcibly adds hydrogen atoms to unsaturated oils (the essential fatty acids are unsaturated oils), making them more saturated and able to postpone rancidity for months. This gives the oil a long shelf-life. Also, hydrogenated oils are more solid at room temperature, so hydrogenation can transform cheap oils into something spreadable. The margarine so created is gussied up with yellow dye to look like butter, for a fraction of butter's cost. *Thus, hydrogenation is an incredibly profitable process for the edible oil industry – who then advertise margarine as though it were good for the heart!*

In fact, researchers have known for thirty years or more that margarine can raise cholesterol and make essential fatty acid deficiencies worse in laboratory animals*. Recently this effect was confirmed in humans, and the researchers concluded in the prestigious *New England Journal of Medicine* that margarine's effects are 'at least as unfavorable as that of cholesterol-raising saturated fatty acids, because they not only raise LDL ['bad'] cholesterol but also lower HDL ['good'] cholesterol levels'[9].

## Margarine Causes Heart Attacks?

Heart attack victims have been found at autopsy to have more hydrogenated fat and less animal fat in their bodies than people who died from other causes[10]. This means that it is likely that these unfortunate people probably did their best to *avoid* cholesterol and *protect* themselves from heart disease by switching from butter to hydrogenated margarine!

The heart attack death rate in different countries varies directly with the amount of essential linoleic acid (from vegetable oils) in body fat. The one-third fall in the American heart-death rate since 1968 was accompanied by a one-third rise in body-fat linoleic acid, following the US public health campaign promoting vegetable oils over animal fat (see page 160). There was no such campaign in the UK, and no such fall in heart attacks. In fact, the UK heart attack rate remains among the highest in the world.

In 1920, there were virtually no heart attacks in America, although *atherosclerosis* was as widespread then as it is now.

*For example, see R. Holman et al., 'Effects of trans Fatty Acid Isomers upon Essential Fatty Acid Deficiency in Rats', P.S.E.B.M., 93:175-179 (1960). Amazingly, researchers seemed to go to any lengths after this to *not* find margarines harmful for humans. One study design had subjects eating a diet very rich in essential fatty acids for weeks (which would tend to build up their reserves) before they were given hydrogenated fats, which, not surprisingly, had little effect on them (F. Matson et al., 'Effect of Hydrogenated Fat on the Plasma Cholesterol and Triglyceride Level of Man', *The American Journal of Clinical Nutrition*, 1975, 28:726-731). That this study was funded by Procter and Gamble, a major margarine manufacturer, is, perhaps, also not surprising.

Then, during the Depression years, hydrogenated margarines and cooking fats took over the market from more expensive butter, and by 1950, over 80% of heart deaths were from heart attacks. The introduction of margarine was the *only* qualitative change in the American diet – and while there was 8% more saturated fat in the 1950 U.S. diet than there was in 1909, there was also *38%* more linoleic acid![11]*

I doubt that this was due to chance! The day that I put together graphs of heart attacks and margarine consumption in America and saw how closely the curves matched (see page 166), I threw out all the margarine in my fridge! Since a working prostaglandin metabolism appears to lower cholesterol naturally, *there is no health reason to use margarine.* In fact, elevated cholesterol in the blood may even be the body's way of *encouraging* the manufacture of more cholesterol-lowering prostaglandins, since the essential fatty acids are transported in the bloodstream attached to cholesterol.

## Cover Up?

Unfortunately, a great many existing studies on the effects of hydrogenates on health were funded by the edible oil industry, and are flawed by bias in their research methods. They were clearly designed to avoid harmful effects by, for example, prefeeding essential fatty acids to crowd out the hydrogenates.[12] Or the experimental period was kept so short that there simply wasn't time for bad effects to surface. But the cleverest ruse of all involved the choice of experimental animal.

Rats and mice – animals often used for these biased studies – have completely different essential fatty acid requirements from us primates, needing far less of the omega-3s. It took a long time for me to spot this, but there are studies which show without any shadow of doubt that monkeys develop the same problems as humans (bad mood, indigestion, poor skin) when they're fed low-omega-3 diets, diets on which rats and mice could live happily ever after.

*A high linoleic acid diet is strongly protective against heart attacks, so it is likely that *nothing* can protect against margarine.

American researcher Dr Donald Rudin concludes from these experiments that, as a population, we are suffering from the same complaint as the omega-3-deprived monkeys, which he has called the 'new pellagra'. We don't all develop the three 'd's' of pellagra (dermatitis, dementia and diarrhoea) at the same time, but vast numbers of us get these symptoms individually, just like the deprived monkeys.

Pellagra is the vitamin $B_3$-deficiency disease, and $B_3$ is vital for the essential fatty acid-to-prostaglandin pathway (page 47). Rudin believes that $B_3$ deficiency inhibits prostaglandin production and caused pellagra's triad of symptoms. He reasons that an essential fatty acid deficiency at a time when we have sufficient $B_3$ will cause less severe prostaglandin shortages and give rise to mild forms of one of pellagra's symptoms. In other words, we should get a kind of group pellagra – which is exactly what we have.

Television advertisements are convincing evidence of this, for most prime-time pitches are for over-the-counter remedies for just three conditions. Skin diseases from acne to itching, digestive difficulties (such as indigestion, haemorrhoids, constipation and irritable bowel), and mood disorders like irritability, depression and PMT (for which we take pain-killers) are epidemic amongst us.

## READ THE LABEL

You've probably got the message by now that hydrogenates are bad for you, but how can you steer clear of them? The chances are that products with long shelf-lives like biscuits, cake mix and potato crisps are loaded with them. There's only one way you can find out for sure – *read the label*! Any product with a label which includes the words 'hydrogenated' or 'partially hydrogenated' will not support your health.

On the other hand, it is important to keep our sense of proportion. I'm not saying you should never eat another chocolate digestive biscuit! Just keep hydrogenate-containing foods to a low level in your diet so that their unhealthful effects are drowned out by the other good stuff you're eating – after all, this strategy protected the laboratory animals in those biased studies!

## Hydrogenation Fosters Essential Fatty Acid Deficiency

Unfortunately, polyunsaturated oils are especially vulnerable to damage from hydrogenation. Almost as a side effect, hydrogenation has an appalling effect on essential fatty acids, changing those it doesn't destroy from the natural **cis** form – in which the molecules are shaped like Js – to **trans** forms*, which are shaped like Is. The true disaster of hydrogenation is that these straighter, trans-form essential fatty acids are worthless as essential fatty acids – prostaglandins cannot be made from them, and they can only be burned for calories. And unlike natural saturates like butter, trans fats actually make essential fatty acid deficiency symptoms worse by getting in the way of the essential fatty acid pathway enzymes, so they act as 'anti-essential fatty acids'. On average, about 14% of fat in the national diet is in the trans form.

When trans essential fatty acids are incorporated into cell membranes, the membranes lose flexibility because the straighter trans molecules pack closer together, reducing red blood cells' ability to squeeze through tight capillaries and lessening the cell-killing effectiveness of white immune-system cells. German researcher Dr Johanna Budwig has shown that the straighter trans molecules allow less oxygen, and more pollutants, through the membrane into the cell. Budwig has almost single-handedly so raised the European consciousness of trans fats that certified trans-free products are now available in Germany and Holland.

Incredibly, American and UK authorities include trans fatty acids in estimating our essential fatty acid intake, reckoned to be 5–10% of calories. A true estimate must reduce this by the 14% of trans essential fatty acids, and then by another 14% to account for the trans fats' 'anti-essential fatty acid' effect. This leaves 4–7%, which is below the American National Research Council's recommendation of 8–10% of calories as essential linoleic acid.

It is even more amazing that this clear and present health danger

*'cis' and 'trans' locate the hydrogen atoms at the double bonds between carbon atoms of the essential fatty acid's skeleton; 'cis' means 'on the same side, and 'trans' means across. Since hydrogen atoms repel each other, a 'cis' bond is bent and a 'trans' bond is straight.

is being ignored, even as the links between essential fatty acid deficiency and heart disease – our number one killer – are strengthening daily.

### Can Essential Fatty Acids Control Overweight?

Besides reducing the risk of heart attack, plenty of essential linoleic acid (from vegetable oils) in your body fat means that you are unlikely to be overweight. This is perhaps not surprising, since overweight is a risk factor for heart disease, but it certainly surprised Dr Peter Oster when he discovered the effect in 650 German citizens[13].

It seems likely that certain 1-prostaglandins activate 'brown fat', a special kind of fat which surrounds and protects vital organs, and which can burn up excess calories[14]. Dr Oster's research suggests that the more essential fatty acids you contain, the more brown-fat-activating prostaglandins you can make, and therefore the more food you can eat without getting fat, since the body's only alternative to burning up excess calories is to deposit them in unsightly bulges around the hips and tummy. Everybody seems to knows at least one lucky thin person with an enormous appetite, and the reason is probably their active brown fat.

Interestingly, babies' appetites increase enormously when they're fed formulas deficient in essential fatty acids, and return to normal on essential fatty acid-rich breast milk[15]. Obviously, babies are immune to the power of suggestion, so this result can't be dismissed as a placebo effect. It seems to prove, rather, that a low essential fatty acid diet sends the appetite out of control. Breast-feeding may even protect against later obesity by laying down stores of essential fatty acids.

## 4. Have No More Than One Egg and One Glass of Milk A Day

Everyone knows that milk is good for you. After all, milk supplies calcium, which builds strong bones and teeth. Most of us get a warm feeling when we think of milk, the legacy of millions of Milk Marketing Board advertisements and comforting childhood milky drinks at bedtime. However, even though it does contain valuable protein, vitamins and minerals, milk may not be quite the panacea it's made out to be.

Amazingly, all over the Western world, the more milk is drunk, the more people suffer from osteoporosis, the crippling bone-loss disease normally associated with calcium *deficiency*. Epidemiologists* discovered this strong association in their studies of diseases in different populations whenever they plotted, for example, hip fractures against milk consumption in the Western nations. No-one is really sure why this should be so, not even the American Dairy Council has managed to show that drinking milk increases the amount of calcium retained in the bodies of adults, in spite of an enormous research effort. The research in this area leads inevitably to the conclusion that milk is not a good source of calcium for adults, in spite of all the advertising trying to persuade us otherwise.

Milk is also linked to heart disease in the Western nations. Antibodies to heated milk proteins are much more common in heart attack victims, showing that their immune systems treated milk as an enemy! Many believe that feeding cow's milk in the first few months of life, before the infant's digestion can properly cope with it, causes this.

Another reason may involve the *homogenization* which makes fat globules in milk smaller so they stay suspended in the milk instead of rising to the surface. Milk contains 'xanthine oxidase', an enzyme which can damage the lining of the arteries and which is one of the many candidates for the agent which causes the initial damage to the arteries in heart disease. In raw milk, this is not a problem, but the smaller fat globules in homogenized milk can be absorbed intact, escaping normal digestion and allowing the xanthine oxidase contained in them to reach the bloodstream. Boiling destroys xanthine oxidase, although this step would not be needed if unpasteurized, unhomogenized milk were widely available.

Many, especially black and Asian people, have a genetic intolerance of milk and lack the enzyme *lactase* necessary to digest

*Epidemiologists study the spread, prevention and control of disease in communities.

the milk sugar *lactose.* A surprising number of juvenile delinquents drink milk in very large amounts, which suggests some sort of craving or food allergy connection.

Milk and eggs both contain saturated fats and plentiful arachidonic acid or AA, which can give rise to the undesirable prostaglandins which constrict the blood vessels and excite the blood to clot if the essential fatty acid pathway is not working properly.

Eggs contain abundant cholesterol, but egg producers have found that feeding fish oils to chickens lowers the amount of cholesterol in their eggs. Free-range chickens get a great deal more essential fatty acids because their diets include insects and green leaves. Since prostaglandins regulate cholesterol levels, free-range eggs are probably much safer for anyone with a tendency towards high cholesterol. It's worth making the effort to find a source of free-range eggs near you, and limiting yourself to one egg a day.

## 5. Buy Organic Vegetables and Fruit and Eat Them Uncooked Whenever Possible

When some people hear phrases like 'organically grown' and 'raw', they tend to think of hippies in communes living on nuts and twigs. I'm certainly not suggesting you eat all your food raw, or try to entertain your dinner guests with nothing but mountainous salads. But if you can manage to work as much raw fruit and vegetables into your daily diet as possible, you'll find the benefits impressive. And if they can be organically grown as well, so much the better.

The reasons behind this suggestion are compelling. There's a long European tradition of natural healing which relies on such foods. And consider Dr Weston Price's 'primitives' with perfect teeth – everything they ate was organically grown, and much of it was uncooked. The fact is, we, as a race, are probably better adapted to raw, organically grown vegetables than to any other food.

The human race ate raw food for almost all its evolution. When cooking was discovered, it vastly increased the range of foods that could be eaten, by, for example, neutralizing toxic enzyme inhibitors in beans, and by killing parasites. This meant that humans could eat almost any local fauna or flora, and so were free to roam, unlike animals constrained to remain wherever their food grew or lived. Thus, cooking may be part of the reason why the human race came to dominate other species and spread out over so much of the globe.

However, cooking also has its disadvantages. For instance, it can actually stop you from losing weight. This is because it breaks down fibre, lessening the fibre content of the diet and interfering with the natural hunger-satisfaction signals which control appetite. It's very hard to eat too much raw food, however, because raw vegetables require more chewing, which also stimulates more saliva for better digestion. Raw vegetables also require more energy for digestion, and *fewer calories are available from them**. All this means is that it's easier to put on weight eating a diet that consists mainly of cooked foods. When Dr John Douglass surveyed more than 200 people eating raw diets in the Los Angeles area, he found *none* who were overweight[16]. This is all the more remarkable because population statistics suggest that such a group should contain more than 70 overweight people.

Should you need any more convincing, consider the following case history. After childbirth, F. couldn't seem to lose the weight she'd gained during pregnancy. Her walk became ungainly, and to many she appeared to have become middle-aged while still in her twenties. However, after just three months of a largely-raw diet combined with an exercise programme, she'd lost some 20

*G. A. Dunayevsky, 'Raw-Eating as a Method of Obesity Treatment', Vrachebnoe Delo, 10:88-91, (1982). Russian language, English abstract: 'Results are reported of treatment of 67 patients with alimentary-metabolic form of obesity associated with hypertensive and ischaemic disease, chronic cholecystitis. The diet consisted mainly of raw vegetable products. A treatment course of 21-24 days resulted in a reduction of the body weight by 10.9 kg or 12% of the initial body weight. The arterial pressure normalized in all patients, electrocardiographic values and those of the lipid metabolism improved. Advantages of this method are absence of complications and its employment in out-patient conditions.' This was interesting enough for me to get the paper translated. Dunayevski checked out the calories available from raw foods and found them much lower than those from the same foods cooked.

pounds, regained her figure and developed a new, slinky-smooth walk. F. is, of course, Fergie, the Duchess of York!

Cooking also destroys vitamins in food, and minerals are discarded with cooking water, so cooked food is less nutritious. And cooked foods apparently separate into layers during digestion, exposing the stomach lining to greater acidity, which can hurt it. Well-chewed raw foods, however, form a porridge-like mass in your stomach which protects the stomach lining.

Along with the loss of fibre, vitamins and minerals, the delicious smells and tastes created during cooking come from a reaction between sugars and amino acids which consumes critically short essential amino acids (such as lysine) in foods. All eight essential amino acids (meaning amino acids which can't be made out of other amino acids, and which therefore must be included in the diet) need to be present for the body to make protein. The leftover, unusable amino acids are burned for calories, which is a messy business and hard on the kidneys.

Cooking reduces the availability of protein in another way. The heat of cooking rearranges some proteins until they cannot be broken down by our digestive enzymes. Even worse, these indigestible proteins then carry digestive enzymes out of the body with them. This means that the pancreas has to make new digestive enzymes – which are themselves made from protein. In other words, *cooking creates a lot of extra work for the body*.

Cooking as much as we do exacts a price we can't afford, and the meals we're used to – a small salad followed by fish with vegetables, for example – is so wildly overbalanced towards protein and cooked vegetables that the few lettuce leaves in the salad can hardly be expected to compensate. What you need instead are large salads full of crunchy vegetables, which form at least three-quarters of the whole meal and which take fifteen minutes to eat.

Once you get the hang of it, such salads are amazingly easy to arrange. Carrots and celery can be taken to the office with a dip. Many restaurants are pleased (if baffled) to give you your vegetables cut up in the usual way, but uncooked, and coleslaw is often available as a side-dish. Sometimes, a decent-sized salad can be made from two or three starters from the hors-d'oeuvres section of the menu.

All the time, bear in mind that the occasional fibre-free, cooked-to-the-limit meal won't do you much harm. Chomping your way through massive salads during power lunches leaves little opportunity to speak, and this may ruin the impression you wish to create!

## ORGANIC IS BEST

At home, your salads should, if possible, be composed of organic vegetables because modern agriculture produces food dangerously low in trace minerals.

Supermarket vegetables seem so depleted of nutrients that you want to back them up with a multivitamin pill – although the study that shows supermarket vegetables plus a multivitamin pill are the equivalent of organically grown vegetables has yet to be performed. Organically grown vegetables, on the other hand, have a successful history of use stretching back to the origin of the human race.

Organically grown vegetables are more expensive, and may not be easy to find unless you live next door to a health food shop. However, more and more health food shops are springing up, and some vegetables are even available through the post. Remember also that local groceries have many suppliers, one of whom may well be able to supply organic vegetables – it's possible that you have only to make your wishes known.

In any case, by asking, you'll be telling the grocer that there's a demand. Satisfying such demands is what makes capitalism work. Your enlightened self-interest can change the face of society, and may even help save the environment by lessening the use of chemical fertilizers and pesticides.

Certified organic growers in California numbered over 400 in 1988, up by nearly 30% since 1987. Certification is an expensive, three-year commitment, and these figures underline the fact that farmers are changing their ways because of public demand. A similar pattern is emerging in Britain with the growing influence of the Soil Association and the Organic Farmers and Growers Association.

*Make no mistake – voting in the marketplace is one of the most powerful statements you can make.*

## 6. Cut Down on Sugar, Refined Flour, Alcohol and Caffeine

I'm sympathetic to the fact that, for most of you, this suggestion embraces all the things that you most enjoy. All I'm proposing, however, is that you try to cut them back, and there are ways to do this without pain. Of course, these recommendations for a healthy diet are well-known to most people by now. They've been endorsed by almost every health authority since they were made in the McGovern 'Dietary Goals for the United States' report way back in 1976, despite howls of protest from the food industry.

These 'foods' all inflame the stomach, elevate stomach acid and/or deplete our bodies of important vitamins and minerals. An inflamed digestive tract allows food fragments into the bloodstream. Retaining their antigenic character (meaning their identity marker proteins remain intact), these drive the immune system crazy, causing food allergies.

Prostaglandin E1 stops inflammation, and Canadian researcher Dr Charles Bates has found that Cytotec (a prescription drug used for treating ulcers which contains synthetic prostaglandin E1) together with evening primrose oil lessens food allergies, and, oddly enough, hangovers. This may mean that much of a hangover's unpleasantness is actually due to food allergy-type effects caused by alcohol's tendency to inflame the digestive tract.

My own allergic foods include milk and coffee. Too much milk triggered sinus headaches, and I had to make a conscious decision to stop drinking coffee because it upset my blood sugar. This was hard at first, until I found that my craving for capuccinos was much easier to control when I started taking *Efamol.*

I had little desire to stop until I realized that, where milky coffee was concerned, I was addicted in the literal sense of the word, '*attached by one's own act*'. I've since found that, contrary to expectation, many people enjoy their allergenic foods in this way. A person's favourite, most frequently eaten food is very likely to be the food that caused their difficulties. Since food allergy symptoms usually don't happen for several hours after the food is eaten, the guilty food is often difficult to spot. However, it's worth making the effort to identify and eliminate them because, over the long-term, I believe they can seriously undermine health. (More on how to do this in Chapter 5, under 'Food Allergy'.)

It's surprisingly easy to do away with sugar. For example, artificial sweeteners like aspartame (in NutraSweet and Canderel) are almost certainly healthier than sugar, although the sugar industry would have you believe otherwise. Sugar-free, all-fruit jams such as the 'Whole Earth' line actually taste better to me than the sugared varieties. A dollop of unsweetened apple sauce tastes great on porridge. And you'll quickly find that the less sugar you eat, the less your sweet tooth will prompt you to eat.

Coffee and alcohol both act as diuretics in the body, increasing the loss of minerals such as zinc and magnesium. Over ninety per cent of us don't get enough zinc in our diets, and almost half of us get insufficient magnesium because of food refining, and because fertilizers don't return enough minerals to the soil. Refined foods like sugar and white flour are 'empty calories' which need more minerals and vitamins for their use by the body than they supply, thus making any existing deficiencies even worse. *Unfortunately, both zinc and magnesium are vital for the 'delicate first step' in processing the essential fatty acids into prostaglandins*, as you can see from the diagram which follows.

## Mineral Deficiencies Are Important!

If you get a cold, your doctor may well prescribe an antihistamine, but rarely recommends zinc lozenges, which can help by boosting your immune response. Most people are terribly short of zinc, but doctors aren't tuned in to mineral deficiencies as contributing factors in illness. You can find out if you're deficient in zinc with 'Check Zinc', a simple test kit available at chemists and health food shops.

Subclinical mineral deficiencies are serious and widespread, but rather than turn this section into a lengthy catalogue of deficiency effects, we'll just take a quick look at magnesium.

During evolution, the diet of the human race was rich in

magnesium and poor in calcium, so the body learned to conserve calcium and store it in the skeleton against a rainy day. But we have no such storage mechanism, and so we need to consume it daily[17].

Although only 39% of actual diets lack sufficient magnesium, most people are deficient because of a failure to absorb enough of the mineral, and because of accelerated depletion. For example, phosphorus from soft drinks binds magnesium in the bowel and prevents its absorption, and calcium supplementation reduces

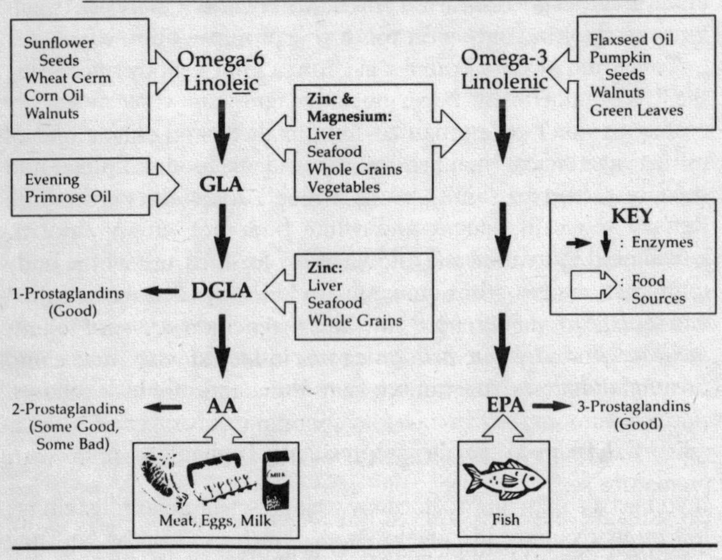


*Figure 2 Minerals necessary for Prostaglandin Production*

*Zinc and magnesium must be present for the 'delicate first step' in which linoleic acid is converted to GLA. Further, zinc is vital for the step in which prostaglandin E1 is created. Calcium (not shown) may also be required, while excess copper (not shown) can inhibit the conversion of DGLA to AA. Unfortunately, food refining has so depleted zinc and magnesium in foods that many of us are deficient in them.*

magnesium uptake. Stress, exercise and drugs (including antibiotics, diuretics and the heart medication digitalis) all increase losses. The upshot is that 80–90% of people wind up deficient in magnesium, according to Mildred Seelig, director of the American College of Nutrition[18]. This is a catastrophe because magnesium has functions in the body, many mediated by prostaglandins, which make it indispensable.

Magnesium helps calcium absorption and encourages bone formation, combating osteoporosis. Heart muscle is usually very low in magnesium after a heart attack, and supplementation increases post-heart attack survival dramatically. Low magnesium apparently *contributes* to heart attacks, since it causes arrhythmias, skipped beats and constricted coronary arteries. Capillaries also constrict when there's too little magnesium, which can lead to a pasty complexion, cold hands and feet, and, for men, even difficulties in achieving erections!

Magnesium supplementation in animals protects them against salt-induced high blood pressure, and lowers both elevated cholesterol and triglycerides. According to American researcher Dr Guy Abraham, who developed the *Optivite* PMT supplement, low magnesium causes the calcification of soft tissues which leads to premature ageing of organs. In the blood vessels, this is called 'hardening of the arteries', while in the kidneys, magnesium deficiency-induced calcification causes kidney stones. By keeping calcium dissolved, magnesium may even assist brain function, since calcium ions are involved in communications between brain cells. Calcification in the brain is definitely associated with premature senility. Indeed, one study showed that old mice fed extra magnesium were able to learn new tasks much more easily than their aged, unsupplemented colleagues.

Low magnesium within cells has even been linked to chronic fatigue syndrome. Apparently, hyperventilation helps compensate for excess acidity within cells, and, when magnesium is low (and acidity therefore high), a complicated feedback loop can perpetuate hyperventilation indefinitely, without the person being aware of it. According to Dr Len McEwan in the *New Scientist*, this causes a feeling of intense fatigue which can be relieved just by teaching proper breathing methods and by taking supplements of magnesium[19]. If you don't think you're tired – don't be too sure! Most people who are *chronically* tired have been that way for so long that they're used to it.

In Germany, magnesium supplements are routinely recommended to pregnant women because they practically eliminate both premature birth and pre-eclampsia, the high blood pressure and fluid-retention malady which affects 5–7% of pregnancies. The Germans consider this so serious that 'failure to take magnesium supplements' is actually included in the list of risk factors for low birth-weight in Germany.

Most of us are more aware of the dangers of calcium deficiency than magnesium, thanks to the advertising efforts of the Milk Marketing Board. But what they don't tell you is that milk has ten times as much calcium as magnesium. This may be just right for calves, but it's catastrophic for humans, who need an entirely different ratio in order for their bodies to efficiently absorb and use calcium. Getting close to the 2:1 magnesium-to-calcium ratio of our evolutionary diet may be a key to avoiding premature ageing, osteoporosis, heart attack and numerous other problems.

Seafood, dark green leafy vegetables and nuts (especially almonds) do contain magnesium, but it's difficult to find enough magnesium in foods. This is one of the reasons I take *Optivite.*

## 7. Take Optivite and Vitamin C

### Take Optivite

*Optivite* is a supplement of zinc, magnesium, vitamins $B_6$, $B_3$, and C with trace minerals and other substances. Although developed to treat PMT, it's a simple way to make sure you're getting the minerals and vitamins needed for the essential fatty acid-to-prostaglandin pathway*. The dose is one *Optivite* per two capsules of *Efamol.*

Like magnesium, pyridoxine ($B_6$) is a problem nutrient[20] – many of us are deficient in it because several aspects of modern

*Does it work? In a trial of *Efavite* (which, like *Optivite,* contains vitamin C, $B_6$, $B_3$, zinc and magnesium), 'there was both greater incorporation of EFAs into red cell membranes and greater clinical improvement in the one month on *Efamol* + *Efavite* than in the four previous months on *Efamol* alone.' From 'Gamma Linolenic Acid', *Reviews in Contemporary Pharmacology,* 1(1):1-41(1990)

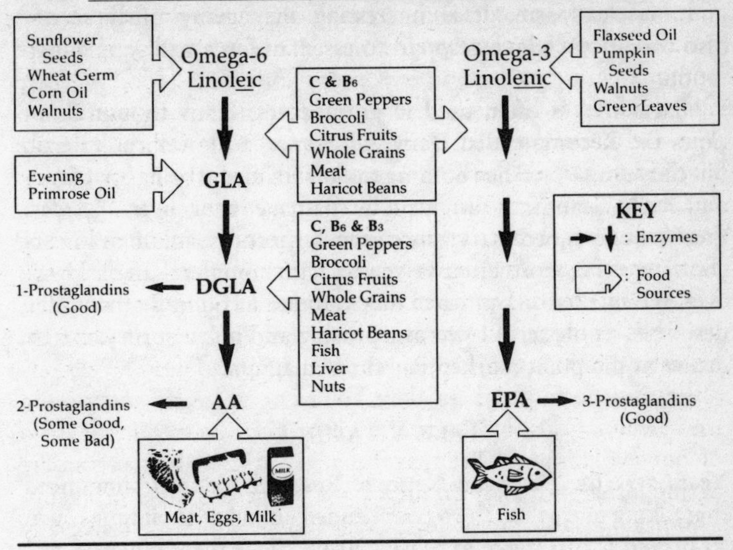


*Figure 3 Vitamins necessary for Prostaglandin Production*

***For prostaglandin production, several 'co-factor' vitamins are necessary: pyridoxine ($B_6$), niacin ($B_3$) and vitamin C assist enzymes at the places indicated in the diagram, and biotin (not shown) is also important. However, as with the mineral co-factors, these nutrients are in short supply in the Western diet because of food refining.***

life cause depletion. For instance, the yellow food dye tartrazine (alias E102) interferes with $B_6$ in the body, and birth control pills, vegetable oils used for cooking and caramel food colouring (E150) are just a few of the things that lower $B_6$ levels in the body.

It seems that $B_6$-depleting factors have been taking their toll, for mild $B_6$ deficiency symptoms such as carpal tunnel syndrome* and the Chinese Restaurant Syndrome[21]** began to appear a few

*Pain or numbness in the hand and wrist.

**Weakness, tingling, headache, light-headedness and/or heartburn after eating monosodium glutamate. Eight of 9 Chinese Restaurant Syndrome victims ceased to react after taking 50 mg of $B_6$ per day for 12 weeks.

decades ago. Other conditions in which low B6 is implicated include tooth decay, hyperactivity, PMT, alcoholism, arthritis and muscle spasm. It is interesting that many of these are also conditions which respond to essential fatty acid supplementation.

Niacin ($B_3$) is often used in gram doses (many thousands of times the Recommended Daily Allowance) to lower cholesterol, but this 'drug effect' has nothing to do with niacin being a vitamin, and such quantities can actually damage your liver. Besides, they're quite unnecessary, since evening primrose oil often lowers cholesterol far more effectively, and with complete safety. However, the smaller quantities of niacin found in *Optivite* encourage desirable, cholesterol-lowering prostaglandin E1 formation by acting at the point marked $B_3$, in the diagram.

## Take Vitamin C

Years ago, the American National Research Council announced that taking more than the recommended amounts of vitamins such as $B_6$ and C just make expensive urine. Since then, however, it's been found that this sort of expensive urine actually protects against bladder cancer!

There are a host of other reasons for taking extra vitamin C. It lessens the frequency and severity of colds, prevents formation of harmful nitrosamines from nitrite food preservatives, arms the white blood cells so that they can zap intruders more effectively and (when taken over many months) lowers cholesterol. Many viral diseases, including viral pneumonia, monocucleosis and chronic fatigue syndrome (nicknamed the yuppie flu) respond to truly heroic doses of 100–200 grams per day*.

Many people believe that any kind of vitamin or mineral 'megadosing' is undesirable and probably harmful. For most vitamins and minerals, this is undoubtedly true. Far too little is known about their long-term effects for anyone to say they are safe to use in such quantities. However, vitamin C produces two effects which suggest to me that we are not getting enough.

The average person's cholesterol level goes up during the

*More on this under 'Chronic Fatigue Syndrome' in Chapter 5.

winter. Doctors are aware of this, and tend to be more conservative about how high a cholesterol level has to be before being classified as 'high' in the winter months. Winter cold is a form of stress, and other stresses can also raise cholesterol levels. For example, all personal tax returns in America are filed on 15 April, and tax accountants as a group are well known to experience high cholesterol during the tax season*. However, vitamin C supplements almost eliminate the cholesterol-elevating effects of both winter and the tax season!

Vitamin C's second effect concerns heart disease. Usually, the cells lining the arteries make 2- and 3-prostaglandins called prostacyclin, which prevents clots from attaching themselves to the wall of the artery, and also lessens the ability of the blood to clot. Where the arterial wall is covered by atherosclerotic plaque, less prostacyclin is made. Extra vitamin C apparently preserved prostacyclin-making capacity until far later in atherosclerosis, which probably lessens heart-attack risk[22].

Another reason for taking supplements of vitamin C is that it helps get rid of the poisons to which our bodies are exposed every day. Several of the body's detoxification schemes use vitamin C[23]. This becomes more and more important as pesticide residues and pollution expose us to greater and greater amounts of chemicals like PCBs which our bodies were never designed to deal with during our evolution as a race.

Vitamin C has never been shown to be harmful**, beyond causing diarrhoea when you take more than you need. There has been a rumour that it causes kidney stones, started by a 1971 editorial in a medical journal[24] which pointed out that vitamin C can cause high oxalic acid (a component of kidney stones) in the urine. *However, no case of kidney stones linked to vitamin C has ever been reported.* In any case, $B_6$ supplementation lowers

*Recently, British men facing the risk of unemployment were found to have higher cholesterol levels than their colleagues whose jobs were safe (*British Medical Journal*, 9.8.90, 301,6750:461)

**However, the *form* in which it is taken is important. Vitamin C is an acid (ascorbic acid), and two grams or more a day causes calcium loss as the body maintains its acid/base balance. Therefore, most authorities suggest taking neutral salts such as calcium, potassium or magnesium ascorbate.

such excessive oxalic acid excretion to normal, suggesting that this effect is actually caused by low $B_6$ levels.

I think of vitamin C as cheap insurance. My three grams or so a day* is derived from a combination of *Optivite* and inexpensive C supplements.

## VITAMIN C AGAINST FREE RADICALS**

It is true that taking pills is a bore, and, to some degree, unnatural. But the fact is, living in today's society subjects us to such unnatural strains and pressures that such measures may be advisable as a kind of backup system to the diet.

One of vitamin C's properties is that it is an antioxidant, capable of neutralizing dangerous free radicals generated by many of the body's processes, such as the 'burning' of glucose for energy in cells. Free radicals are also made during the detoxification of poisonous chemicals*** in the liver. One reason why they are so incredibly destructive is that each free radical reaction generates a new free radical – like a fire, free radical reactions can feed on themselves. Left un-neutralized, free radicals damage vital biological structures such as our DNA genetic material, and cause the cross-linking which colours age spots and wrinkles the skin. Supple animal skin is turned to leather by this same free radical process.

## ARE YOU CROSS-LINKED?

Take the 'pinch test' to find out if your skin is ageing faster than you are. Pull up a pinch of skin from the back of your hand for five seconds and then release it. Count the number of seconds it takes for the mark to disappear. If the number of seconds is greater than your age in decades, watch out!

*Remember, I'm diabetic. Vitamin C transport is insulin-dependent, so diabetics may need more.

**Free radicals are molecular fragments with unpaired electrons which are attracted to hydrogen ions so strongly that they will actually tear apart other molecules to get them.

***Including substances we don't usually think of as toxic, such as the acetaminophen in headache remedies.

## Free Radical Protection

Preventing free radical reactions is important to the body, since it maintains an intricate and interdependent network of antioxidant defences in which selenium*, vitamin E, vitamin C and beta-carotene are front-line soldiers. For example, strategically placed molecules of vitamin E in cell membranes stop free radical reactions from tearing through the membrane, leaving trails of destruction behind them. The antioxidant nutrients also protect against cancer, and help the immune system to do its job. Pollution, food additives, drugs (prescription and otherwise), exercise, second-hand cigarette smoke and stress all increase your need for these nutrients, so making sure that you get plenty is just common sense.

According to Dr Denham Harman of the University of Nebraska College of Medicine, controlling free radicals reduces the rate at which we age[25]. One study showed that supplements of C and E reduced the rate at which body fat becomes rancid (a free radical reaction) by 25%. This is enormously encouraging because less rancidity means less lipofuscin (the pigment which colours liver spots) and younger, better-looking skin. It also means more artery-lubricating protective prostacyclins, since prostacyclin formation is inhibited by rancid fats in the bloodstream.

Omega-3 fish oils are protected against rancidity while they remain in the fish, but are very prone to react with oxygen and become rancid as soon as they're extracted. The cod liver oil many of us took against our will as children for its A and D content had an extremely unpleasant taste, caused by rancidity.

However, taking fish oil supplements apparently increases vitamin E requirements many times (seventeen times in one rat experiment), and may interfere with vitamin E absorption.

Antioxidants also inhibit the release of arachidonic acid (AA)

*Selenium seems to work closely with vitamin E. Natural sources include Brazil nuts, salmon, tuna, swordfish, crustaceans, whole grains and sunflower seeds. Low selenium apparently contributes to cancer (*Cancer Res.* 49(21):6144 and *J. Nat. Cancer Inst.*, 82(10):864), digestive diseases (*J. Int. Med.*, 225:85) and asthma, since those with low selenium-containing glutathione peroxidase had *five times* the asthma risk (*Clinical Science*, 77(5):495 and *Thorax*, 45:95).

from membrane storage – remember, AA is the omega-6 fatty acid found in meat, from which the undesirable 2-prostaglandins are made. Less AA release means that there are fewer unwanted 2-prostaglandins to cause the blood to clot and obstruct the blood vessels – just what the doctor ordered!

## 8. Take Fibre Supplements

***Big stools, little hospitals. Little stools, big hospitals.***

Denis Burkitt, MD

***Eat bran and the world will fall out of your bottom.***

Graffiti

Food processing has reduced the fibre content of our food to dangerous levels. Although the ***Food for Vitality*** programme does supply more fibre in the form of whole grains, vegetables and fruit, it's silly to expect that everyone who reads this book will make radical dietary changes overnight. In the interim, and for those days when you slip off the Plan, a fibre supplement makes sense. Such supplements can control both constipation and diarrhoea, and make life infinitely more pleasant for those who suffer from haemorrhoids.

Low fibre diets go hand in hand with constipation, ulcers, diverticular disease, gall stones, polyps, irritable bowel syndrome, tooth decay, haemorrhoids, appendicitis, varicose veins and even deep-vein phlebitis, the disease which nearly killed President Nixon*. One reason for this is mechanical: the bowels need bulk to work properly. Soluble fibres absorb many times their own weight in water and add bulk to the stool. This allows rapid movement of food through the gut, which denies bacteria the chance to break bile down into cancer-causing carcinogens and also lessens the time irritants remain in contact with the bowel wall. Hence, fibre may also protect against cancer.

Fibre lowers cholesterol by carrying bile out of the body. Bile is made in the liver, and emulsifies fats in the digestive tract so they can be digested. Since bile is formed from cholesterol, cholesterol must be withdrawn from the blood to make more,

*From T.L. Cleave, *The Saccharine Disease*, Keats, New Canaan CT, 1975

thus lowering the amount left to cause trouble in your arteries. Oat bran is often hailed as a cholesterol reducer, and, interestingly, oat bran also contains some cholesterol-lowering GLA[26].

Of course, a disturbed essential fatty acid-to-prostaglandin pathway is the original cause of high cholesterol*, as Dr David Horrobin's studies with evening primrose oil have demonstrated. Thus, it's no coincidence that the nutrients which aid reactions in the essential fatty acid-to-prostaglandin pathway (zinc, magnesium, $B_6$, $B_3$ and C) all have cholesterol-lowering actions. Similarly, the factors which interfere with the pathway (stress, saturated fat, sugar, alcohol and the hydrogenates in margarine) can all raise your cholesterol level.

What kind of fibre supplement should you take? Wheat bran is often advertised, but soluble fibres such as psyllium husks (pronounced 'silly-um' and found in products like Metamucil), guar gum or oat bran provide more protection than insoluble kinds like wheat bran, which can be coarse and irritating. The phytates in insoluble fibre like wheat bran can also completely surround (or chelate) mineral atoms and reduce the amounts of calcium, magnesium, zinc and iron absorbed by the body.

A dessert-spoon a day of psyllium husks is usually about right for impeccable bowel action – *but it's vital to work up to this sort of quantity*. Starting out with too high a dose is a very common error, and *will* cause bloating, belching, stomach-aches and frequent embarrassing noises, so prudence dictates no more than a teaspoon to start with.

## Conclusions

So that's the ***Food for Vitality*** programme in a nutshell. Give it a try! You can expect changes to begin within two weeks of starting the programme, although improvements will continue for many months. While it's not a substitute for medical attention if

*During weight loss, cholesterol may be temporarily elevated – the researchers who found this effect speculate that the extra cholesterol is released from fat cells ('Weight Down, Cholesterol Up?' *In Health Magazine*, September 1991)

you're ill, there's every likelihood that eating this way will greatly reduce illness in your life. Some enlightened doctors actually prescribe programmes very like this one to speed recovery, and hundreds of people have successfully used this and closely similar programmes to improve their health.

There's one final point that I'd like to make. I realize that the people reading this book will be as diverse as the stars in the sky. You come in all shapes and sizes – men, women, home-makers, pilots and candle-stick makers. But all of you in your own way want to improve your lot and start embracing change.

The ***Food for Vitality*** approach is a different idea, based on the premise that the body is important – a living, breathing machine whose condition determines how you feel. I never used to think of my body this way. I used to be proud of my 'cast-iron' digestion, and that my body seemed able to take anything I could throw at it – even as I stared into the mirror at the reflection of a balding man shaped like a Bartlett pear.

Believing that the condition of the body is at the core of one's sense of well-being is, for many, a new idea. It's a big change to grasp that connection, and it means hard work. It's frightening to think of remaking ourselves – but the rewards are wonderful. When we decide to stop our self-destructive behaviour and take positive steps to change, we feel the first stirrings, very strange, of deserved self-respect coming from a completely new source. When I did it, at first I didn't recognize this new person – but it was me.

> ***In the midst of winter***
> ***I found within me***
> ***An invincible summer***
> ALBERT CAMUS

What can make this possible for you is your new knowledge of the prostaglandins' effects. Acting on this knowledge truly sets you free – free from the cravings which interfere with your appetite. It also makes you immune to television pitches from advertising agencies, who are only too happy to promote any product as 'healthful' – whatever its effect on your body. Food processors aren't in it for your health, though. Why should they be? The only person who *really* has a stake in that is you. But now you and they are on a more even footing.

I want to feel better. I want to get as much out of life as I can. I want to live as long as possible in robust health, and sign out of this life with that good feeling that comes after a day well-spent. Does this sound naive? Well, what's wrong with that? Someone recently asked the painter Robert Rauschenberg if he still saw things through a child's eyes. 'Yes,' he said, 'I'm totally naive. Do you know how much effort it takes to be 64 and naive?' Rauschenberg knows how important it is to retain a fresh and child-like view of the world, however old you are. And that includes being constantly receptive to new ideas. I think that my ***Food for Vitality*** programme helps me maintain such an attitude – feeling young, fit and strong in spite of being middle-aged is a wonderful antidote to cynicism and misanthropy.

We can all improve the quality of our lives, enjoy happier relationships, be more fulfilled and spend more of our lives at the peak of our abilities than perhaps any generation which has gone before. It's an exciting prospect.

Now let us see how all this came to be.

# 3: Eat, Drink And Be Wary

This is a detective story. *Something* is killing us before our time. Clues abound in our patterns of illness, and on our plates. Many have tried to solve this 'murder mystery', but until now science couldn't supply the forensic evidence needed to break the case. Although some of the following may seem heavy going, stay tuned. Everything comes out all right and there's happy endings for all – except the perpetrators.

## Innocent Victims

The elephants in the National Wildlife Park near Murchison Falls in the Protectorate of Uganda were losing their health, but when conservationists established the 2,000 square-mile Park as a tourist attraction, their future seemed assured. The elephants prospered. They knocked down some trees to reach the succulent upper leaves, stripped the bark from others (which kills the tree) and ate the rapidly-growing young bushes in between with gusto. Such normal, healthy elephant carryings-on help to maintain a good mixture of forest, scrub and grassland in the wild. However, in the limited area of the Park, the slower-growing shrubs and trees had little chance to grow back and gradually areas of open grassland grew.

Eventually, in spite of the plentiful rich grass, the elephants' health declined. They developed hardening of the arteries, lessened fertility, increased infant mortality and stunted growth.

Research revealed that the elephants lacked linoleic acid, an essential fatty acid vital for the health of their arteries*. The natural environment of elephants is woodland, and a large area of woodland is required to support a single elephant. Over-population was destroying their habitat so that their natural diet was no longer available to them.

The solution was to shoot them until their numbers no longer overwhelmed the environment, which seems particularly cruel because their plight was no fault of their own. Also elephants seem so wise and benevolent, and their family groups mirror the bonds of affection which exist in human families.

That we humans are in a similar predicament (although for different reasons) was not really brought home to me until I read about these elephants. The millions of rats who have given their lives in laboratories the world over demonstrating similar things somehow don't translate into human terms, and just don't have the same impact.

However, we are deteriorating in our own way, and this is shown only too clearly by our heart attacks, child abuse, soccer hooliganism, inner city despair, our children's declining ability to learn, rampant drug and alcohol abuse and the rising incidence of premature senility and Alzheimer's disease.

Incredibly, with all our medical knowledge, our life-expectancy at 50 years of age is only a couple of years longer than in 1841!** Our *average lifespan* has increased greatly because fewer babies die, not because we're living any longer. It's as though something is working against our great advances – something which reduces our lifespan even as better medicine and better nutrition lengthen it.

We have learnt to transplant hearts and decode our genes, but we still don't know why so many of us have heart attacks or die with our minds addled! Our brains are our highest specialization, the thing which distinguishes us from other forms of life, and they, too, are deteriorating! Can we use them to solve this problem? In fact, since there are no benevolent elephants to shoot us, we must solve it or perish.

*Grasses contain plentiful LNA (linolenic acid) but little of the LA (linoleic acid) – which elephants get from the leaves, bark and seeds of trees.

**1980 statistics.

Can it have to do with what we eat? The evidence is slim (even if many of us are not), for our health problems don't respond dramatically to dietary improvements. However, the evidence looks much stronger if you take a longer view.

## *Pottenger's Cats*

Dr Francis Pottenger's ten-year study of cats eating various diets over several generations is unique in medical literature[1]*.

Cats fed raw meat, milk and cod liver oil maintained broad faces and regular teeth through the generations, showing striking uniformity in size and skeletal development with lustrous fur and little shedding. They were resistant to infections, parasites and allergies, and were, in general, gregarious, friendly and predictable in behaviour. Miscarriages were rare, and mother cats nursed their young without difficulty.

In contrast, cats fed scraps from the Pottenger Sanitarium differed widely amongst themselves after only one generation. After three generations, their narrowed skulls and smaller jaws showed crowded teeth. Other skeletal changes included lower calcium levels with longer, thinner bones and narrower pelvises. Their coats were also rougher with numerous skin problems.

Pottenger wrote that 'they develop all kinds of allergies. They sneeze, wheeze and scratch. They are irritable, nervous and do not purr. Healthy first-generation cats fed scraps produce second-generation kittens with allergies, and by the third generation, the incidence is almost 100 per cent**.' Parasites and infections were common, along with heart problems, near- and far-sightedness, arthritis and hypothyroidism***.

Pregnant females frequently aborted; deliveries were difficult, with many deaths during labour. The kittens weighed nearly 20% less than those of the healthy group, and showed high infant

*Dr Pottenger treated conditions like asthma with adrenal extracts, and he standardized the strength of these extracts by feeding them to cats.

**Francis M. Pottenger, *Pottenger's Cats*. Published by and available from the Price-Pottenger Nutrition Foundation, PO Box 2614, La Mesa, CA 92044-2614, USA. Tel. (714) 582 4168

***Too little thyroid hormone causes weight gain, fatigue, dry skin, constipation, arthritis and a slowing of bodily processes.

mortality. As to mood, the females were irritable, some to the extent of being dangerous to handle, while the males were more passive and showed abnormal sexual activity.

So far, there are actually few surprises. We know that poor nutrition can cause all sorts of problems, so health failure in poorly fed cats is not remarkable. However, the thing that stands out is that all the problems became worse with each passing generation, and, most importantly, *it took four generations for depleted cats to become healthy once more when they were returned to their natural diet.*

## Healthy Teeth

If diet was really important, so the argument goes, it would have an unmistakable effect on disease. However, if Pottenger's effect holds true in people, then a chronic illness may have its beginnings in, say, a grandmother's alcoholism and be compounded by a mother's poor diet. It's hardly fair to expect such a condition, several generations in the making, to be cured by a few dietary changes late in life.

But *does* Pottenger's effect hold true in people? Much evidence suggests that it does. Dr Weston Price, a contemporary of Dr Pottenger's, published *Nutrition and Physical Degeneration: A Comparison of Primitive and Modern Diets and Their Effects* in 1939[2]. He found the diets of fourteen primitive cultures from around the world, including North and South American Indians, isolated mountain Swiss, Gaelics, Eskimos, Melanesians, Polynesians, Aborigines, Malays, Maoris and tribes of Eastern and Central Africa, to be far more nutritious than the 'civilized' diet of his day.

Remarkably, all fourteen groups had virtually perfect teeth on their traditional diets, but developed rampant decay as soon as they adopted modern refined foods – indeed, toothache was the only reason for suicide in some groups. And as with Pottenger's cats, their characteristic broad dental arches gave each a wide face so that the traditional-living people presented a consistent appearance, as though all were members of the same family.

But on Western food their faces became narrower and teeth more crowded with each succeeding generation, giving a more

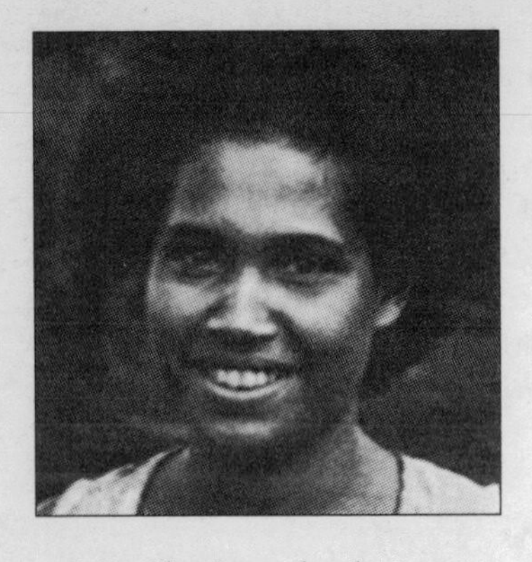

S. Pacific. Bone development determines size and shape of palate and nasal air passages

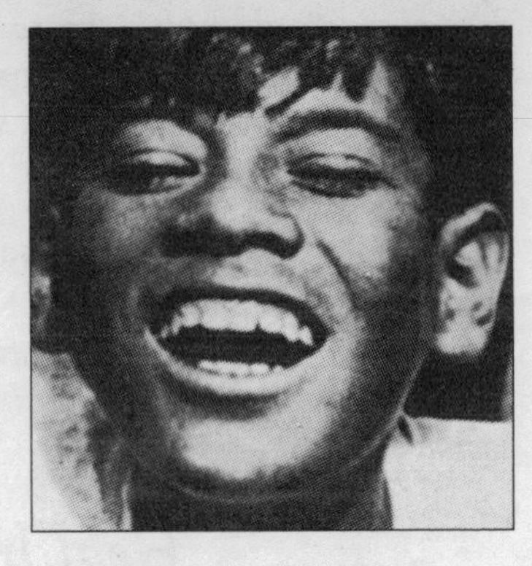

Polynesian with a perfect dental arch

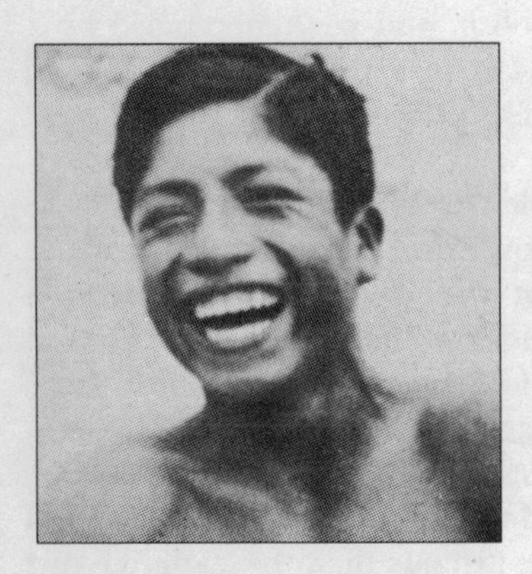

Peruvian fisherman. Note breadth of dental arch and development of facial bones

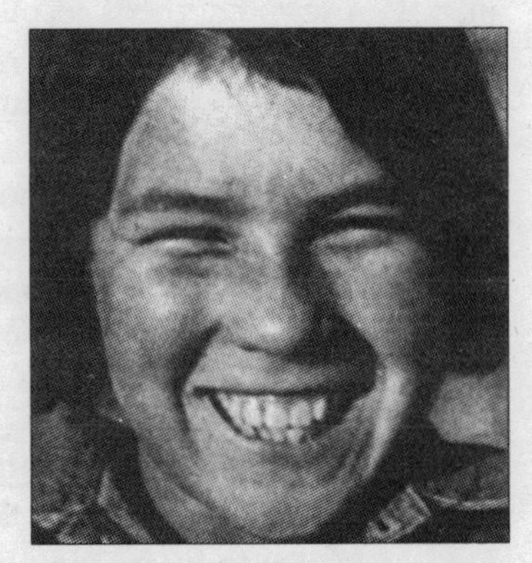

Alaskan Eskimo. Broad face with a broad dental arch and no tooth decay

***Figure 4** Dr Weston Price's illustrations of people eating traditional diets produce the same broad dental arches and fully-developed facial bones elsewhere. Used with permission.*

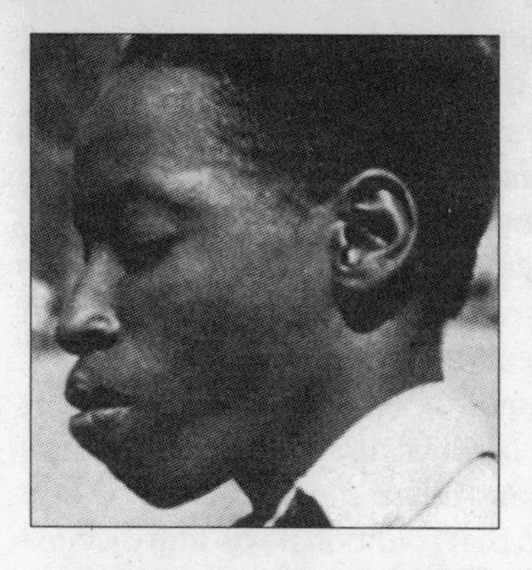

Short lower jaw one generation after modern food arrived in Nairobi

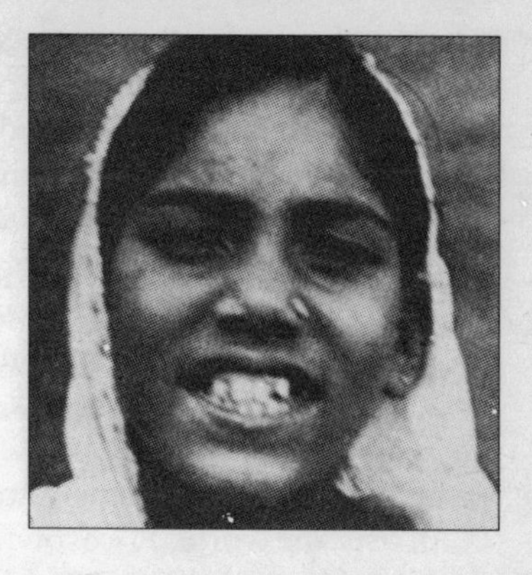

Cairo. Typical face and dental arch injury *is not limited to visual stucture*

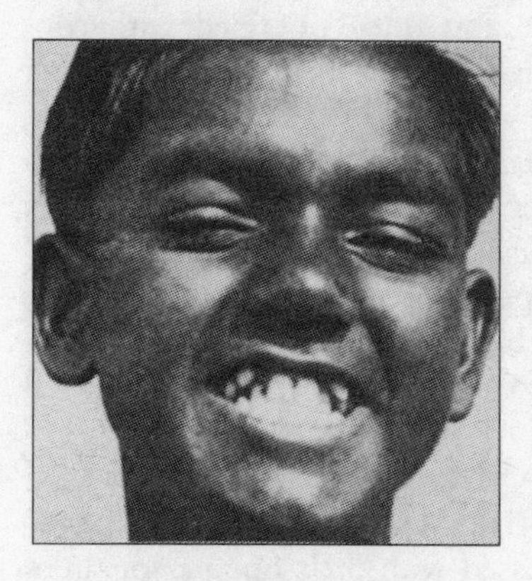

European look in a child whose parents have typical African racial characteristics

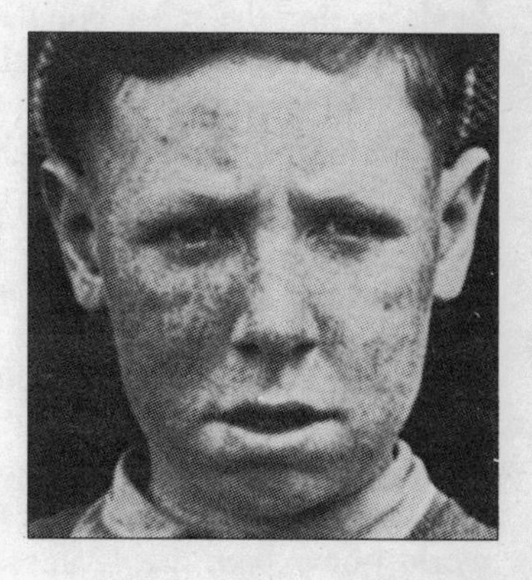

Alaskan white with narrow nostrils and crowded teeth. A mouth-breather

*Figure 5 Dr Weston Price's illustrations of people eating refined foods. 'Modernization has produced a sad wreckage of physique and often character . . . These faces are stamped with the blight which so many think of as normal because it is so common with us.' Weston Price, DDS. Used with permission.*

varied individual appearance. Sinus problems, mouth-breathing, pinched nostrils, poor vision, troublesome wisdom teeth and, extraordinarily, a rarity of good singing voices resulted. Price was amazed at the number of magnificent potential operatic tenors he encountered amongst the traditional-living peoples on his travels.

Similarly, an increase in height accompanied by a narrowing of the body caused difficulties in childbirth for women. Such problems were almost unknown among traditional-living peoples, as an Eskimo woman's remark indicates: when she gave birth at night she didn't bother to wake her husband sleeping beside her, rather waiting until morning to introduce the new child.

All over the world, Price found that traditional wisdom dictated the use of some rich source of 'fat-soluble factors' for preventing tooth decay and producing 'a human stock of high vitality'. Such foods included sea life, animal organ meats or dairy products from animals raised on rapidly growing spring grass*, with sea foods by far the most popular and often obtained with considerable difficulty. He even found dried fish eggs and kelp high in the Andes mountains!

Primitive peoples paid much attention to nutrition in pregnancy. Even before conception, potential mothers and even fathers were often fed special foods, usually seafoods. Some cultures' social constraints provided for spaced pregnancies, a practice that we are discovering minimizes birth defects. The result was a uniformly high standard of nutrition, with benefits going well beyond those already listed.

For example, Price found sunny dispositions: 'As I sojourned among members of primitive racial stocks in several parts of the world I have been deeply impressed with their fine personalities and strong characters . . . Fundamentally, they are spiritual and have a devout reverence for an all-powerful, all-pervading power which not only protects and provides for them, but accepts them as a part of that great encompassing soul if they obey nature's laws . . . few impressions can be more vivid than their absence

*Sea foods were by far the most effective diet. The number of decayed teeth among the Swiss Alps population who used the dairy products was almost five per cent, while the seafood groups were well below one half of one per cent. Now, *there's* an unmistakable effect of diet on disease!

of prisons and asylums. Few, if any, of the problems which confront modern civilization are more serious and disturbing than the progressive increase in the percentage of individuals with unsocial traits and a lack of responsibility. For the two thousand inhabitants [of the until-recently isolated Loeschental Valley in Switzerland] there is no prison. In Uganda, Africa, the Ruanda tribe estimated to number two-and-a-half millions has no prisons.'

As Pottenger observed in his cats, Weston Price saw in people a breakdown in immunity and an increase in antisocial tendencies, accompanied by characteristic changes in appearance* on inadequate diets. Price noticed that in every case where modern refined food became available to traditional-living peoples, the younger members switched to them in spite of their elders' pointing out what it was doing to them. In other words, *there is something profoundly addictive about inadequate nutrition.*

So why do modern diets disturb our appetites and make us irritable and prone to disease and dental decay? Price discovered low levels of vitamins and minerals in the modern diets of his day, but surely these shortcomings have been corrected in today's diet? After all, we don't have scurvy, rickets or pellagra.

Price probably didn't know his 'fat soluble factors' included the then newly discovered essential fatty acids (EFAs). But, nonetheless, our health apparently depends on our ability to obtain and use these essential oils.

## *The Plot Thickens*

Further clues are to be found in *The Driving Force*** by Dr Michael Crawford and David Marsh. They point out that body tissues contain fats and oils in roughly dietary proportions, so that the ratio of omega-6 (land) and omega-3 (sea) oils in human

*This effect is so reliable that it has even been used to distinguish the fossil remains of domestic dogs from wolves – 'Within a few generations of breeding in captivity, the facial region of the skull and jaws becomes shortened, this being common in many species but is most apparent in early domestic dogs . . . this causes a crowding [of the teeth]' (J. Clutton-Brock, *Domesticated Animals from Early Times*, British Museum of Natural History, 1981).

**William Heinemann Ltd., UK, 1989

and cod liver is about 3:1 and 1:22, respectively, but *the brains of both human and cod have the same 1:1 percentage of essential fatty acids, regardless of species.*

Nearly half the dry weight of the brains of whales, dolphins, rats, apes and man are essential fatty acid derivatives, about evenly divided between the two families of essential fatty acids, the omega-3s and omega-6s. On land, LA (linoleic acid, parent of the omega-6 group) is plentiful in nuts and seeds (and, hence, in vegetable oils), while green leaves supply quite small amounts of LNA (linolenic acid), forebear of the omega-3 family.

Grazing animals laboriously convert these into useful derivatives, which carnivores acquire from them ready-made. In fact, many of the cat family cannot convert the EFAs at all, and quickly sicken when they are withheld. This was one reason why big cats in zoos failed to breed when fed on EFA-poor muscle meats. When they make a kill in the wild, they eat the EFA-rich liver, heart, kidneys and lungs first, followed by the ribs for calcium*.

In the ocean, it is the other way around: omega-6 oils are hard to find but the omega-3 derivatives EPA and DHA** are readily available from plankton at the bottom of the food chain. So it is all the more surprising that the brains of fish and men are virtually identical in composition – there is, apparently, only one way to make a brain.

The intriguing thing about Crawford's observation is that we survive with only about 1% of calories as omega-3 oils in our diet, despite our most valuable tissues being dependent upon them. We have a superb adaptation to low dietary levels, and we've been pushing it to the limit – beyond the limit, in fact.

It's no wonder that Weston Price found primitive peoples far from the ocean preparing for pregnancy with seafoods! And perhaps this explains in part why perinatal malnutrition stunts the child's IQ, for if the raw materials are not there during the

*So your cat's prescription should include chicken livers and mackerel. My cat Dennis recovered from feline acne when I added chicken livers to his diet.

**Remember – omega-6 (seed oils): LA→GLA→DGLA→AA, forms PGE1 ('good'), PGE2 ('bad')
– omega-3 (fish oils): LNA→EPA→DHA, forms PGE3 ('good')
– the fats in the brain are largely AA and DHA.

critical period of brain development, then the brain must be less than it could be*.

Human breast milk is so rich in EFA derivatives that a six-month-old infant gets the equivalent of six ounces of chicken livers or two-and-a-half ounces of sheep's brains a day!** To put it another way, a breast-fed infant gets the equivalent of 3–4 capsules of *Efamol* evening primrose oil. In contrast, cow's milk is designed to nurture a large-bodied, small-brained calf and contains but one-sixth of the EFA amount in human milk. At two years of age, a calf's brain is about 0.2% of its body weight, while the figure for a human infant is a whopping 8%!

Are bottle-fed infants at a disadvantage? Experiments on rats have tried to answer this question. A low-EFA diet for rat mothers during breast-feeding resulted in learning deficits in the pups[3]; and when litters of pups were redistributed, the pups of mothers with many to feed had small brains, while small litters made for large brains[4]. And in another experiment, there were lowered brain cell counts by the third generation of rats fed a low essential-fatty-acid diet[5] – and here again is the theme of a progressive decline over several generations that Pottenger saw in his cats***.

Apparently, mothers' IQs predict how well-fed their babies are, and a low IQ often means a malnourished baby****. This stunts

*Anything but human breast milk probably fosters malnutrition because a baby's EFA reserves are marginal at birth (R.T. Holman et al., 'Effect of Sex and Age on Fatty Acid Composition of Human Lipids', *Am. J. Clinical Nutrition*, 1979, 32:2390-99).

**Human colostrum: 8% LA, 0.3% GLA, 0.3% DGLA; human breast milk: 11% LA, 0.4% GLA, 0.3% DGLA (R. Gibson et al., *Am. J. Clin. Nutr.* 1981, 34:252-257).

***It is very ominous in this connection that the brain of a domesticated sheep is 30% smaller than that of a wild species of about the same size (M. Crawford and D. Marsh, *The Driving Force*. William Heinemann Ltd., UK, 1989). Are we in danger of losing our brains?

****You'd think this would have more to do with the mother's knowledge of nutrition, but while this is undoubtedly also a predictor, low maternal IQ was found to correlate with maternal and infant IQ, and 'those affected are limited, making it difficult for them to be wholly incorporated in [society]' and prone to childhood elevation of cholesterol and blood pressure. (J.W. Prescott et al., *Brain Function and Malnutrition*, John Wiley & Sons, N.Y., 1975, quoted in M. Crawford, *The Driving Force*, William Heinemann Ltd., 1989).

the child's intellectual development, producing an adult who contributes less to society – and who is likely to feed his or her own children poorly.

This 'cycle of deprivation' means that birth defects and educational abnormality are much higher in lower socio-economic groups. The effect is so pronounced that simply giving an ordinary multi-vitamin pill to high-risk mothers cuts birth defects by 85%![6]

The blood vessels which nourish the heart require many of the same nutrients as the brain. Hence, low IQ, low birth weight and *increased risk of stroke and heart attack later in life* all go together[7].

## Heart Attack, Anyone?

A fascinating study of 1500 Canadian infants who died accidentally from various causes (other than heart disease) found early signs of atherosclerosis* to be seven times as frequent in bottle-fed as compared to breast-fed babies[8]. The cholesterol levels of Western children begin to be elevated over those of African children at 6–8 years of age[9]. The researchers pointed out that since the children are unlikely to be smoking**, heart disease probably begins early in life, and is made worse by lifelong dietary shortcomings. It's not really surprising therefore that *half* of 105 American soldiers aged about 22 years had atherosclerosis when they were killed in Vietnam[10].

As long ago as 1956, Dr Hugh Sinclair found that the body easily transports cholesterol linoleate, which is made from cholesterol and linoleic acid[11]. But if LA is in short supply, cholesterol oleate (made of cholesterol and oleic acid – olive oil is mostly oleic acid) gets made instead. And cholesterol oleate is hard to move and gets deposited in all the wrong places.

*Fatty streaks which some believe eventually develop into atherosclerotic plaque.

**Smoking mothers show atherosclerosis in the umbilical cord, and smoking causes low birth weight. Interestingly, smoking also confounded the protective effect of plentiful EFAs in the body fat in a study of Scottish men's proneness to heart attacks.

## *The Messengers*

Plentiful linoleic acid has a cholesterol-lowering effect. However, the linoleic acid derivative prostaglandin E1 apparently instructs the liver to make less cholesterol if there's enough available from food.

### THE CHOLESTEROL BALANCE[12]

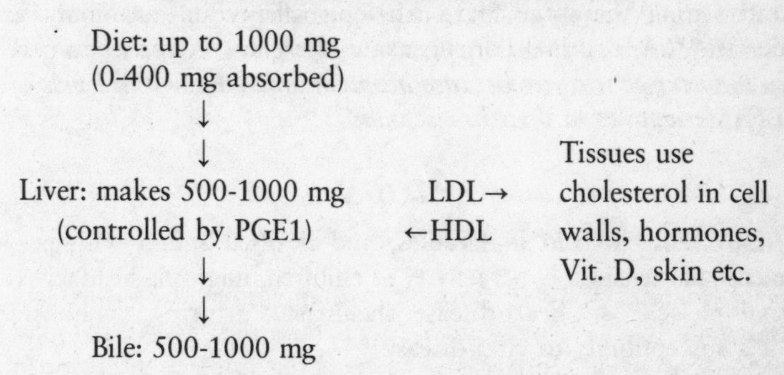


Up to 400 mg of cholesterol absorbed from food adds to the 500-1000 mg made in the liver. Cholesterol is transported to the tissues in the bloodstream as Low Density Lipoprotein (LDL), where it is used to make hormones, cell walls, etc. Any excess comes back to the liver as High Density Lipoprotein (HDL) and is made into bile to help with digestion (more on page 163.) On a low fibre diet, most of the bile is reabsorbed and the cholesterol recycled, but a high fibre diet carries much of it out of the body. Hence, bloodstream cholesterol will build up unless little is eaten, the liver doesn't make very much and a high fibre diet is eaten.

This messenger function is disturbed by poor diet, *but it can be restored by detouring around the blockage.* The GLA in evening primrose oil lowers cholesterol up to 170 times more than the same amount of linoleic acid, which means that evening primrose oil can partially make up for a poor diet and return the control mechanism for cholesterol production to working order.

Other messengers can have catastrophic health effects when disturbed. For example, low essential fatty acids* in umbilical-cord blood, caused by, say, a mother's poor diet, *can cause the foetus's immune system to be over-active.* Certain prostaglandins damp the immune system, and, consequently, low cord-blood EFAs are

*The disturbed pattern is normal LA with low GLA, DGLA and AA.

usually found with an over-active immune system[13]*, meaning the child is likely to suffer from atopy, the inherited tendency to develop allergies. Atopic asthma, eczema and hay fever are surprisingly widespread, affecting one in five of the population.

So we begin to see how Pottenger's cats came to 'sneeze, wheeze and scratch.' Low essential fatty acid derivatives set the thermostat on the kittens' immune systems too high, giving rise to antibodies against harmless things such as pollen or the cat's own skin cells and setting the stage for a life-long allergy or auto-immune disease**. And, just as Pottenger saw, *allergies will likely be worse in the next generation because atopic mothers have low levels of EFA derivatives in their breast milk*[14].

## Atopy

Atopy tends to run in families, and is often found with premenstrual tension, hyperactivity in children, migraine headaches, multiple sclerosis, heart disease, rheumatoid arthritis, alcoholism or a susceptibility to viral diseases***.

*Indicated by high levels of immunoglobulin E antibodies.

**It may also be that the tissues are imperfectly formed – after all, EFAs form a large part of the skin, mucous membranes, vascular and nervous system. If the appropriate EFA derivatives aren't to be found, then the developing foetus must substitute or perish. Thus, poorly formed myelin has been put forward as the reason that the immune system attacks nervous tissue in Multiple Sclerosis, since the EFA processing enzymes make components of myelin.

***Multiple Sclerosis follows the distribution of heart disease (R.L. Swank et al., 'Multiple Sclerosis: The Lipid Relationship', *Am. J. Clin. Nutr.,* 1988, 48:1387-1393), and those with PMT are likely to have an atopic background (A. Atton-Chamala et al., 'Premenstrual syndrome and atopy: a double-blind clinical evaluation of treatment with a gamma-globulin/histamine complex', *Pharmatherapeutica,* 1980, 2(7):481-486). People with atopic eczema are abnormally vulnerable to viral diseases, and the viral diseases Epstein Barr and AIDs sometimes trigger atopy (*Omega-6 EFAs,* D. Horrobin, ed., Wiley Liss, 1990, p.36) Most hyperactive children have atopic families, and 'atopy is common in patients with ulcerative colitis, Crohn's disease, ear problems, nasal polyps and some obstetric problems.' (Judy Graham, *Evening Primrose Oil,* Thorsons, 1988). 'Cystic Fibrosis is a disease which is believed to be due to an enzyme abnormality fully expressed only in homozygous patients. Heterozygous carriers of cystic fibrosis are frequently phenotypically atopic (from M.S. Manku, 'EFA levels in the Plasma of Patients with Atopic Eczema' in *Clinical Uses of the Essential Fatty Acids,* ed. D.F. Horrobin, Eden Press, 1982; J.O. Warner et al., 'Cystic Fibrosis Heterozygosity in the Pathogenesis of Allergy', *Lancet,* 1976, 1:980)

An atopic family might have an alcoholic grandfather, a mother with PMT, a hyperactive child whose sisters have eczema, asthma and hay fever, and an uncle with blinding headaches and sore knees. Sufferers from this cluster of diseases have one thing in common: *low blood levels of the EFA derivatives.*

## *Low EFA Derivatives in Diseases*

Most EFA processing takes place in the liver, and tissues which can't process the EFAs (such as the skin) are supplied with derivatives through the bloodstream. Other tissues, like the platelets and white cells of the blood, can make their own.

However, if there aren't enough essential fatty acids during a child's critical period of development, then it seems that the enzyme machinery never really works properly – as in atopy. As a consequence, each of the atopic group of diseases seems to have a unique pattern of deficiencies in specific tissues. For example, in atopic asthma, EFA derivatives are normal in plasma but deficient in white blood cells, while in atopic eczema they are deficient in both.

Other conditions inhibit the EFA metabolism. In diabetes, high blood sugar and low insulin both affect the first of the EFA-processing enzymes. Race is also a factor, for a northern coastal ancestry means a weaker enzyme system to start with, and age eventually undermines even the strongest system. A poor diet can do the same thing – Dr Donald Rudin investigated the changes in the American diet over the last hundred years and found that[15]:

1. Omega-3s are down 80%
2. B-vitamins are down 50%
3. Vitamin $B_6$ may be low in almost everyone because of milling, which has also reduced fibre by 75 to 80%
4. The antioxidants vitamin E and selenium are down for the same reason, selenium by more than 50%
5. Antinutrients have increased substantially – saturated fat is up

by 100%, cholesterol by 50%, refined sugar by nearly 1000%, salt by 500%, and trans fats from hydrogenated fats by 1000%

These inadequacies can themselves cause a pattern of low EFA derivatives which, in turn, may cause atopy in the next generation. Such a pattern also makes ailments such as PMT more likely, and predisposes to alcoholism, migraine, heart attack*, rheumatoid arthritis and so forth. Let's call this Pottenger's effect.

Normal levels of the essential fatty acids and their derivatives are remarkably stable in healthy people the world over, apparently another example of homeostasis, the body's control of internal conditions. The graph opposite compares the patterns of omega-6 essential fatty acid derivatives** in diabetics, alcoholics and sufferers from PMT and atopic eczema (which have very similar patterns) with normal levels.

In these diseases, something is clearly wrong with the enzyme which converts the linoleic acid found in seed oils to GLA, so that PGE1 and other prostaglandins must be lower than normal. But lessened PGE1 paradoxically means *more* inflammatory 2-prostaglandins from AA (in spite of lowered AA levels)[16], so *this disturbed pattern is associated with increased inflammation and elevated auto-immunity.* This means more clotting and arterial spasm so that a heart attack becomes more likely, and will predispose to allergic conditions and diseases such as arthritis.

Alcoholics apparently prefer food low in linoleic acid*** or absorb it poorly, for their LA level is lower than normal, and this compounds their enzyme problem.

Diabetics and those with PMT and atopic eczema evidently

*LA and most polyunsaturated acids, including AA and EPA, were lower in [heart attack victims] . . . The fatty acid pattern of serum phospholipids is an independent risk factor for coronary heart disease ('Fatty-acid Composition of Serum Lipids Predicts Myocardial Infarction', *Brit. Med. J.*, 9 Oct., 1982, 285:993).

**Specifically, in the plasma phospholipid fraction, which contains the most essential fatty acids. Levels in this fraction are fairly stable, unlike the free fatty acids, cholesterol esters and triglycerides which change with each meal.

***Is this why bacon and eggs is a popular breakfast among the hungover?

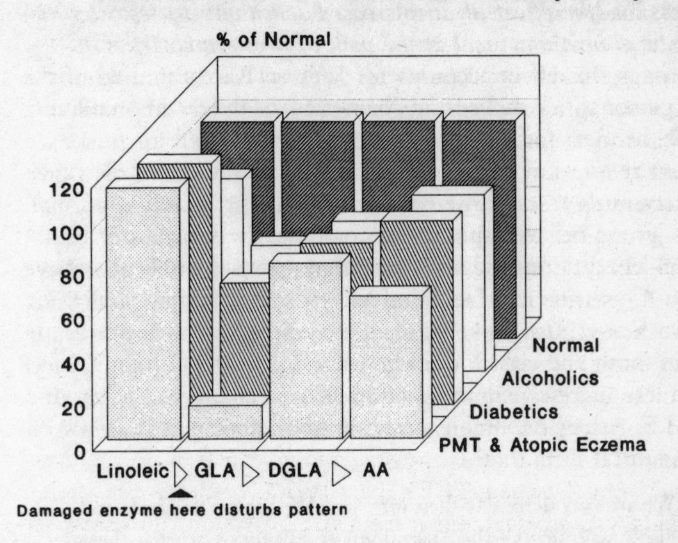


*Figure 6 Patterns of Disturbed Essential Fatty Acids in Illness*

*These distorted patterns of EFA derivatives have serious health effects. Low DGLA means low prostaglandin E1, so heart attacks, irritability and cancer become more likely. Arachidonic acid (AA) is a key component of the brain, nervous system and blood vessels, so chronic low levels means these tissues must deteriorate.*

have ample LA but impaired capacity to convert it*. In PMT, low EFAs in cell membranes seem to make cells over-sensitive to normal levels of oestrogen and progesterone, for the terrible moods of PMT can be produced in normal women by giving them extra hormones. But this begs the question: what is the corresponding effect in men?

*Remember that DGLA is formed from LA via GLA, and the PGE1 formed from DGLA thins the blood and improves the mood.

If men have three times the EFA requirement of women, and three-quarters of women have PMT, *then a heightening of aggression* (*the effect of an increased sensitivity to testosterone*) *must be almost universal in the men of Western societies.*

Perhaps this effect accounts for Weston Price's finding of the 'fine personalities and strong characters' of the traditional-living people he met, and for their apparent lack of need for prisons.

If we're *all* more aggressive because of our Western diet, then we may jump to the false conclusion that aggression is normal. Thus, Freud believed that the id could barely contain our brutal animal legacy, Konrad Lorenz held that man is innately aggressive in *On Aggression* and Desmond Morris said much the same thing in *The Naked Ape.* Have we slandered ourselves? Is nature really 'red in tooth and claw'* or *only when necessary*? Certainly, I feel much less aggressive than I used to before I changed my diet, and Dr M.F. Ashley-Montagu wrote of Aborigines and Eskimos on their natural diets that:

> We are very definitely their inferiors. We lisp noble ideals and noble sentiments – the Australians and Eskimos practice them – they neither write books nor lecture about them. Theirs are the only true democracies where every individual finds his happiness in catering to the happiness of the group, and where anyone who in any way threatens the welfare of the group is dealt with as an abnormality**.

The American anthropologist Ashley Montagu (no relation) wrote that 'aggressiveness is taught, as are all forms of violence which human beings exhibit . . . Aggression is the expression of the frustrated expectation of love.' I firmly believe this, for it is entirely consistent with the insights of so many of my patients about their own aggression.

Now it's time for more forensic evidence in the case of the

*Very little activity in nature is pointless, for those who do not waste energy have more with which to ensure their survival.

**Quoted in W.A. Price, *Nutrition and Physical Degeneration*, Price-Pottenger Foundation, La Mesa, CA, 1982

disturbed EFA derivatives. We have got to crack this case because we are in the same boat as the elephants. We, too, are deteriorating because we're not getting the essential fatty acids we need, and in our run-down state, we are also heedlessly destroying our environment, over-populating it far beyond its carrying capacity and failing to husband its resources. Many are starving in the third world, as well. The parallel is uncomfortably close.

# 4: Getting Better

The crime has now been reconstructed in our 'murder mystery'. It's clear that noxious influences disturb the patterns of essential fatty acid derivatives in a cluster of seemingly unrelated diseases. What is to be done? Can these patterns be corrected and, if so, does it make any difference?

*When the diet of diabetics with nerve damage was supplemented with eight capsules of GLA-rich evening primrose oil per day, their disturbed patterns of essential fatty acid derivatives moved towards normal*[1]. *With this change, the diabetics' neuropathies improved.*

The figure opposite shows the changes in the levels of GLA, DGLA and AA, and, as can be seen, the supplement largely corrected the effect of the malfunctioning enzyme. DGLA is back to normal.

Similarly, in alcoholics, evening primrose oil reduced Valium use during withdrawal and improved liver and brain function (especially those skills needed for driving). *No previous treatment (other than $B_1$ supplementation) has ever had a positive effect on brain function*[2].

And several studies have shown that both atopic eczema and PMT improve with evening primrose oil supplementation. In other words, evening primrose oil both corrects the distorted patterns of EFA derivatives in, and also improves, all four conditions. There is every likelihood that it will do the same in any of the raft of diseases connected with such distorted patterns. *Hence, those of us who are likely to show such a pattern, whether*

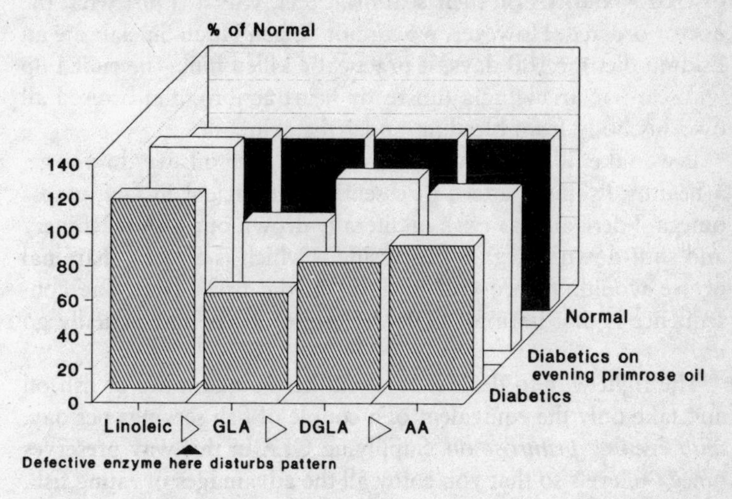


*Figure 7 Effect of Efamol on Patterns of Disturbed Essential Fatty Acids*

***Notice how the evening primrose oil corrects the diabetic pattern. DGLA is back to normal and AA is almost normal once more. The diabetics' neuropathies improved markedly with these changes.***

*from ageing, viral infections, illness or the Pottenger effect, are well advised to consider taking evening primrose oil.*

Of course, a good diet is the first line of defence. Every supplement under the sun cannot make a poor diet equivalent to the pattern of eating described in Chapter 2, and supplementation will be far more effective as part of a diet free of excess saturated fat, refined foods, hydrogenates and foods you're addicted to.

## *Surely, Fish Oil's Better?*

Mega-dosing on fish oil is fashionable today. Some argue that as the Eskimos don't have heart attacks, neither will we if we eat like Eskimos. There's only one thing wrong with this – *Eskimos* *are different from us.* In a superb example of adaptation to an extreme diet, Eskimos lack both the 'delicate first step' enzyme, and the enzyme which makes AA*. They can sustain healthy levels of DGLA and AA on their seal-meat diet, which is just what the doctor ordered. However, we cannot. When Hugh Sinclair ate an Eskimo diet for 100 days, it practically killed him – he ended up with cardiac arrhythmia (unsteady heart action), and bruised all over his body from bleeding under the skin.

If we take 30-gram megadoses of cod liver oil, we do *not* get a healthy Eskimo-pattern of essential fatty acids! In fact, excess omega-3 derivatives in fish oil literally drown our EFA machinery and shut down omega-6 processing – which is already marginal or we wouldn't need cod liver oil in the first place. The consequence is that harmful LDL cholesterol levels may actually go *up*.

The right way to do it is to avoid heroic quantities of fish oil and take only the equivalent of a couple of fish servings per day, *with evening primrose oil.* Supplying GLA in this way preserves omega-6 levels so that you enjoy all the advantages of eating fish, such as lower triglycerides and a reduced risk of heart attack, as well as lowered LDL cholesterol. The *combination* produces the healthful Eskimo blood picture.

## Omega-3s are not a Panacea

The current fish oil hysteria really is over the top. Our omega-6 requirement is close to *six times* our need for the omega-3s**, for this is the ratio in most of our tissues. It is easy to induce omega-6 deficiency symptoms, but depriving somebody of omega-3s seems to have little effect. In fact, omega-3 supplementation when omega-6 derivatives are low actually *brings on* deficiency symptoms because the omega-3s inhibit processing of whatever omega-6 is available. We need *both* families of essential fatty acids in the

*The missing enzymes are delta 6-desaturase and delta 5-desaturase, which are the same enzymes missing in cats. Hugh Sinclair called Eskimos 'obligate carnivores', acknowledging that they have to obtain all their EFA derivatives from their diet.

**Except during pregnancy and breast-feeding, when omega-3 requirements are higher during development of the omega-3 rich brain and retina.

roughly 6:1 proportion that we've grown used to over millions of years.

## Why Evening Primrose Oil?

Evening primrose oil is considerably more expensive than other sources of GLA, but it has been used in most clinical trials, so that its good effects have been demonstrated. The same is not true of other sources.

But surely, you say, GLA is GLA, and the beneficial effect of any supplement must be related to the amount of GLA in the oil? Not so, apparently. In experiments to discover the best source of GLA, Dr David Horrobin compared evening primrose oil with blackcurrant seed oil, borage seed oil and fungus oil. He found that blackcurrant seed oil actually *increased* levels of inflammatory thromboxanes by five times. Fungal oil halved output of PGE1, and simultaneously cut beneficial prostacyclin output by a third. And blackcurrant and borage seed oils were less than one fifth as effective as primrose oil in boosting PGE1 levels[3]. Perhaps the tiny quantities of unusual oils in other sources inhibit the GLA, or the linoleic acid in evening primrose oil has some good effect.

What is clear is that, in the present state of our knowledge, evening primrose oil is the best bet. In fact, it is prescribed in Finland and the UK for eczema, and used in Japan to make the oils in baby formulas closer to the profile in mother's milk. However, evening primrose *plus* fish gives the best chance of correcting the fatty acid imbalances associated with the diseases that kill us.

## Who Can Be Helped?

Diabetes exaggerates our Western tendency to atherosclerosis by about six times, but Dr Houtsmuller of Rotterdam found lessened complications (including heart attacks) among diabetics on a high-linoleic-acid diet. Dr Houtsmuller's diet supplied so much LA that it probably forced more through the defective enzyme step, which suggests that evening primrose oil will provide even more effective protection against heart attack in those who do not have diabetes, by bypassing the malfunctioning enzyme and supplying protective GLA directly.

Others who may benefit include those with atopy and chronic fatigue syndrome*, those at risk from heart attack or cancer, the aged, drinkers, hyperactive children of atopic families, hypertensives (especially the salt-sensitive) and migraine sufferers, as well as the irritable and depressed. But pregnant mothers have the most to gain, for their children are more likely to be whole and well-adjusted. In fact, preparing for pregnancy as Weston Price's traditional-living peoples did is the best strategy**.

## *Primal Therapy and The Importance of a Good Birth*

In my work as a psychologist, a Primal therapist, I find that birth and what happens soon after has lifelong effects. I know how strange this sounds, but consider these two 1987 studies. 'Perinatal Origin of Adult Self-Destructive Behaviour'[4] described how in 412 Scandinavian suicides, alcoholics and drug addicts, 'suicides involving asphyxiation were closely associated with asphyxia at birth***, suicides by violent means were associated with mechanical birth trauma [forceps, etc.] and drug addiction was associated with opiate and/or barbiturate administration to mothers during labour.' Mothers of alcoholics usually had chloroform anaesthesia, while mothers of hard drug users got opiates or barbiturates.

The second study linked 'Perinatal Distress and Prognosis of Psychotic Illness.'[5] Babies who suffered through a prolonged labour and/or a difficult delivery were far more likely to become schizophrenic, irregardless of their family history****.

It doesn't stop there. Child abuse often lurks behind 'borderline

*Those who recover from an Epstein Barr virus infection but still suffer chronic fatigue were found to have a characteristic pattern of disturbed EFA derivatives, so the Chronic Fatigue Syndrome may be added to the list.

**See under 'Pregnancy' in the next chapter.

***Caused by the umbilical cord being wrapped around the neck of the child during birth.

****A recent study has linked birth trauma to a lower IQ (F.J. Roemer, *Obstetrics and Gynecology*, May 1991).

personality disorders', characterized by intense, unstable relationships, impulsive self-destructive behaviour (such as drug abuse and manipulative suicide attempts), rage alternating with childish dependence on others and feelings of emptiness. Females in this category (which includes about 20% of those who seek psychological help) outnumber males 2.5 to 1, perhaps reflecting the fact that girls are at far more risk of sexual abuse than boys[6]*.

We *all* suffered childhood traumas, so we're all more or less repressed and therefore neurotic. *An often-overlooked consequence of this repression is lowered immunity,* since endorphins**, the agents of repression, dampen natural killer cells' ability to destroy infected or malignant cells[7]***.

Primal theory holds that we suppress consciousness of these traumas to protect ourselves. We may be hardly aware of these memories stored beneath consciousness, but they apparently impel us to constantly re-create the traumas of our childhoods *in order to try to solve them.* This is the repetition compulsion we see everywhere, in our choice of wives or husbands, in the treatment

*A strong literature supports this contention. See L. Salle et al., 'Relationship of Maternal and Perinatal Conditions to Eventual Adolescent Suicide', *Lancet*, 1:624-627 (1985); J. Gray et al., 'Perinatal Complications as Predictors of Developmental Disabilities', *Developmental Neuropsychology*, 5(2-3):105-113 (1989); C. Kopp, 'Risks in Infancy: Appraising the Research', *Merrill-Palmer Quarterly*, 36(1):117-139 (1990); L. Muhlen et al., 'Effects of Type of Birth and Anaesthetic on Neonatal Behavioral Assessment Scale Scores', *Australian Psychologist*, 219(2):253-270 (1986); R. Morrock, 'Birth Symbolism and Batmania', *J. Psychohistory*, 17(2):207-214 (1989); E. Kandel, 'From Metapsychology to Molecular Biology: Explorations Into The Nature of Anxiety', *Am. J. Psychiatry*, 140(10):1277-1293 (1983); R. Fischman et al., 'Long-lasting Effects of Early Barbiturates on Central Nervous System Behaviour', *Neuroscience and Biobehavioural Reviews*, 7:19-28 (1983); J. Wilcox, 'Perinatal Distress and Infectious Diseases as Risk Factors for Catatonia', *Psychopathology*, 19:196-199 (1986); 'Behavioural Teratology: Birth Defects of the Mind', *Science*, 202:732-734 (1978); E. Gemmette, 'Anxiety Associated With Trauma', *Psychological Reports*, 50:942 (1982); G. Aylward et al., 'Correlation of Asphyxia And Other Risk Factors With Outcome: A Contemporary View', *Developmental Medicine and Child Neurology*, 31:329-340 (1989)

**Endorphins are almost certainly generated when we are hopeful and optimistic, so 'hope is dope'. Rudyard Kipling's remark that 'Words are, of course, the most powerful drug used by mankind' embraces this idea.

***A related consequence is that heroin addicts are wide open to infections.

of our children and in our compulsive behaviour (including self-destructive eating patterns). The depression which affects some 80% of us at some point in our lives surely stems from the same source, an *appropriate reaction* to long-past events *displaced in time.*

Such 'Pain' is probably the reason Marilyn Monroe felt unloved in spite of being adored by millions, for nobody in the present can fill the gap left by a parent in the past *until this deprivation is made fully conscious.*

Most people are overtaken by painful childhood memories at some time. A scent, a surprise meeting, returning to childhood neighbourhoods or even events in a film can do it. A trapdoor opens in memory, and one is suddenly *in* some melancholy past event. Proust talks about this in his *Remembrance of Things Past,* and even established psychological theories tacitly acknowledge it. One example holds that 'a person's exposure to a hypercritical or exploitative environment as a child leads to painful, unprocessed feelings that emerge reflexively when the person is exposed to stress later in life.'[8]

Nobel Laureate Albert Szent-Gyorgi remarked that 'discovery consists in seeing what everybody else has seen and thinking what nobody has thought.' In this way, Dr Arthur Janov discovered a systematic way of bringing such trauma to consciousness, resolving both the Pain and the unconscious behaviour it produces*. He found that eliciting details of a painful event brings repressed feelings into consciousness with all their attendant sadness and tears. This *experiencing* allows the memory's integration into consciousness, for, shorn of the emotional overload, it is no longer a threat – and repression is no longer necessary.

For example, I dared not cry when my Father died because my Mother was falling apart and I feared I would lose her too. In therapy, telling him 'goodbye' plunged me into the acute anguish I felt at eight years of age, but could not express. After several months of 'feeling' the impact of his death, my outlook ceased its frequent alternation between irritation and sadness.

Anger mobilized and protected me against the pain of my unmet needs. When this pain threatened to get out of control, I had to

*Arthur Janov, Ph.D., *The New Primal Scream*, Abacus, London, 1991

repress everything and became sad. I had spent much of my life struggling against impulses stemming from unexpressed grief at my bereavement. This mountain of old feelings controlled my life, but once felt, they became just memories. I think this is why there are so few books about Primal Therapy – it is profoundly undramatic to point to an eight-year-old's misery, but discussing the angst, existential doubts and manic-depressive tendencies that result has filled thousands of books.

Talk-therapy such as counselling, encounter groups or psychoanalysis merely increases *awareness* of these past problems, but it is their *experience* which allows the curative integration into consciousness. Conventional wisdom holds that approaches such as Janov's are disintegrative and foster hysteria, but quite the reverse is true.

The repressed memory constantly activates the body to respond to the *old* situation, which is inappropriate, stressful, and, ultimately, exhausting*. After Primal therapy, you are *more* conscious because more of your life's experience is available to you, *and many health and behavioural problems, such as high blood pressure and irritability, are alleviated*[9]**.

How is it that either Primal therapy, dealing with our food allergies (page 151) or improving the fats in our diets result in similar health improvements? I believe that the common factor is that all three approaches lessen stress hormones such as adrenalin and cortisol which can block the 'delicate first step' of the essential fatty acid metabolism***. All three strategies will likely raise PGE1 levels and reduce the 'bad' 2-series prostaglandins.

*The same leakage powers the repetition compulsion. We continually re-create the conditions of our destruction in order to solve them. Unfortunately, the solution must be symbolic, for it leaves the past untouched and unresolved. We therefore remain unsatisfied – and the closer we come to resolution, the worse we feel!

**The world is woefully short of Primal therapists, but Dr Arthur Janov and I are endeavouring to change this at the Primal Training Center in California (2554 Lincoln Blvd., Marina del Rey, CA 90291, USA (213) 392-2003). To be an effective Primal therapist, one must both undergo the process and undertake an intensive training programme, for this learned skill is almost impossible to acquire if impulses from old situations compete with those from the present.

***Stress may also raise inflammatory prostaglandins by promoting a more oxidizing climate in the body. This causes the immune system to become friskier, worsening a whole raft of immune-related problems.

There are some indications that the pattern of disturbed essential fatty acid levels apparently occurs in those whose pain exceeds their capacity for repression*. Certainly, correcting such a pattern provides some relief! In addition to lessening stress hormones, it may be that the right prostaglandins optimize neural receptor function in the brain in the same way that they are thought to modulate our sensitivity to hormones in conditions such as premenstrual tension.

We are far more influenced than we suppose by what happens during our very early development. The well-nourished foetus of a well-nourished mother who is free of pain medication stands an infinitely better chance of making it into this life unscathed. I'm convinced that decent birth practices (including fewer caesarean sections**), breast-feeding and measures such as constant touching for incubator babies would cut our epidemic rate of psychological disturbance in half.

## *Should we Return to our Evolutionary Diet?*

Many people speculate about what we ate during our evolution as land-dwellers. Most assume, with the mainstream anthropologists, that we are savannah creatures, meaning that we came down from the trees into the open plains of Africa and there learned to walk upright and make tools. They argue that our diet

*69% of a group of depressed children came from families with a high rate of both alcoholism and depression (*Science News*, 1989, 136(6):90-91). This link between depression and the disturbed EFA pattern recurs in the findings that hostility (a symptom of major depression) boosted the risk of later death from heart disease by five to seven times (*Science News*, 1989, 136(4):60), and that as many as 33% of heart patients are clinically depressed (*Science News*, 1989, 135(91):13). Dr Charles Bates reports considerable success in alleviating both hostility and depression with evening primrose oil and other measures to normalize the EFA pattern (C. Bates, *Essential Fatty Acids in Immunity and Mental Health*, Life Sciences Press, Tacoma WA, 1987).

**Caesarean section deprives the foetus of the vaginal squeezing during birth which seems to be equivalent to animal mothers' licking of face and perineum after birth. This activates the genito-urinary and gastro-intestinal systems. Puppies die if not licked, and Caesarean-section human infants have more tummy troubles and are harder to comfort than those who are born naturally.

must have included meat, roots, shoots and seeds, and that we will keep our health if we return to a similar pattern of eating[10]. This means, in their opinion, a high-fibre, relatively low-fat diet with plenty of polyunsaturated but little saturated fat, and plenty of complex carbohydrates from vegetables, seeds and fruits. It all seems eminently sensible, but are they right?

In *The Driving Force**, Dr Michael Crawford and David Marsh point out that we have several features which make a savannah origin unlikely. For example, like seals, we have subcutaneous fat and a diving reflex, meaning that the pulse drops when we immerse our heads in water, conserving oxygen. We can, like hippopotamuses, sweat huge quantities of water to control our temperature. We are hairless, like dolphins. And our newborns swim with their eyes open and breathing controlled if they are put in water, although they lose this talent if it is not exercised in the first six months of life.

In contrast, Crawford and Marsh point out that savannah species like antelope do not sweat and have efficient kidneys which minimize urine losses, allowing them to get by on little water. Their hair protects them from the sun and assists in temperature control by trapping a layer of air next to the skin. And *they are uniformly small-brained,* as might be expected from the small quantities of linoleic acid available in their food**. In fact, 'nowhere in the world today is there any evidence of modern man having made any adaptations to the semi-arid savannahs.' Put like that, it strains the credulity that we would have chosen to evolve in such a barren, inhospitable place.

Rather, they suggest, we evolved at the ocean margin, where we would have had the best of both worlds – two ecologies to exploit for food, and plentiful marine omega-3s and omega-6s from land plants to make big brains. We have 'an extraordinarily persistent love of water' and can swim very long distances, such as across the English Channel. It's a telling point that 'the five civilizations to evolve written languages all emerged on rivers or estuaries: the Yangtze, the Ganges, the Indus, the Nile, the Tigris and the Euphrates.'

*Harper & Row, William Heinemann Ltd., London, 1989
**There is plentiful linolenic acid in grasses, but little linoleic acid.

They make a strong case – where would you prefer to live? – and if they're right, our evolutionary diet, like the diet proposed in this book, was very rich in the essential fatty acids.

## *Which Sex?*

As mentioned above, oestrogen and progesterone levels are near normal in PMT, but some believe the body over-reacts to them when the EFA derivatives which control hormonal sensitivity are low in cell membranes.

In the final stages of pregnancy, hormonal changes are thought to trigger the specific reorganization of brain development which determines if the child's outlook will become that of a male. The theory goes that if this does not occur, the child's outlook will be female regardless of whether the body develops as male or female[11]. *If this is so, EFA derivatives modulate the deciding of our sexual identity – and low levels may confuse this process.*

## *The Perpetrator Revealed*

Heart disease. Cancer. Auto-immunity. Low IQ and antisocial tendencies. Alcoholism. Homosexuality. All these may be linked to poor essential fatty acid nutrition.

The question is: *why* is there poor essential fatty acid nutrition? After all, if we aren't getting enough EFAs then we all should have the classic deficiency symptoms: slowed growth, brittle and dull hair, nail problems, dandruff, dermatitis, thirst with strong urine – but we don't.

Rather, it may be that we can't use the EFAs we do get because of the blockages explored in the last chapter: too much non-essential fat, cholesterol, alcohol and hydrogenates; viral infections; and too little C, $B_6$, $B_3$, magnesium and zinc.

But how can this be? Surely (the tabloids scream) you don't mean that the villains are our friends the farmers and food processors, those benevolent magicians who conjure up crisps and pork pies?

You understand (the defence argues) that our exploding population makes cities necessary so that land remains for agriculture, and that food refining and hydrogenation are necessary to give shelf-life so the foods can reach the city?

But (says the prosecution) it seems that food processing for taste without nourishment actually increases our appetites, so food producers intentionally over-refine and then distort our food choices towards their products with advertising – for no other reason than to make a profit. For is it not true that health authorities suggest we put together once more what the food producers have so painstakingly taken apart?

We are urged to spread our white breakfast toast with polyunsaturate-rich margarine, and to take a high-fibre cereal. With a vitamin pill containing the nutrients removed by the miller, we have a pathetic travesty of the nutrition available in wholegrain bread – at many times the expense.

And is it not both usual and profitable, and, unfortunately, also lethal, to add saturated fat to farm animals? How is it that a domestic animal contains a staggering twelve times more calories from fat than its wild cousin? Our farmers' skills are clearly devoted to leaving us badly nourished and craving more of their defective products!*

In closing arguments, the defence throws itself on the mercy of the court: society is to blame. Society *wants* crisps and pork pies. Every one of us has control over what he or she eats, and, further, has control over the money which is exchanged for it in the market place. If the public indicated its desire by diverting money towards more nutritious foods, the entire food industry would rapidly respond**.

But (thunders the Judge) such choices require knowledge denied the average consumer because those caught in the cycle of deprivation are the very people most influenced by advertising, most vulnerable to deficient foods and least able to grasp the arguments advanced here – *because of the deficient foods they have been induced to eat.* Guilty as charged.

*Remember that infants' appetites increase enormously when their formula is deficient in essential fatty acid derivatives.

**Julia Hailes, an author of *The Green Consumer Guide*, remarked that 'if the market demands change, all obstacles people want to put up mean nothing, because whoever gets there first gets the business: it's a very fast way of making things happen.'

The sentence? A slap on the wrist.

If we change to healthy foods overnight, there might be chaos in the marketplace. We don't want food prices to rise, do we? We wouldn't want to shake public confidence in the food supply (particularly after the salmonella and the BSE)? We don't want to bite the hand that feeds us. The Prime Minister wouldn't like it, the Government could fall. So we'll seal the decision and let it join the NACNE report in that uneasy obscurity behind the platitudes of the Ministry of Food and Agriculture, and call it a triumph of political diplomacy.

## *The Population Explosion*

***Human life and turnips remain cheap and plentiful***

FRANK HUBBARD, *1868–1930*

***We come inevitably to the fundamental question: What are people for? What is living for? If the answer is a life of dignity, decency and opportunity, then every increase in population means a decrease in all three.***

MARYA MANNES, *1904–*

But perhaps our exploding population renders all this inconsequential. In 1798, John Malthus pointed out that populations always grow faster than their food supply, and that environmental exhaustion causes a massive die-back whenever populations reach the stage of explosive growth – as ours has. Science and technology may postpone this, but they add pollution and the greenhouse effect to the stresses on the environment and simply postpone the inevitable crisis.

We will need exactly those faculties under the most intense assault to overcome our ancient, blind imperative to go forth and multiply. To stand a ghost of a chance of surviving, we must overturn our religious convictions against birth control, appreciate the compassion of a 'successful famine' and place the health of the environment over our convenience.

Although nailing jelly to the ceiling would be easier, there is one cheering prospect in this dismal picture. *Dietary improvements could bring with them the very attitudes necessary for our survival as a race.*

Weston Price's traditional-living peoples respected their environments, and, before turning to Western foods, would no more have dreamed of the abuses we practise than fly to the moon. After all, the Aborigines lived in harmony with their environment and in population equilibrium for forty thousand years before Captain Cook arrived.

## *Pottenger's Effect in People*

The Japanese are the longest-lived of all industrialized peoples. Interestingly, they also eat the most fish and have a largely wholefood diet with the high ratio of essential to non-essential fatty acids which Sinclair suggests will be healthful.

Traditional-living Japanese are small and broad-faced, with excellent evenly spaced teeth, the hallmarks of Weston Price's healthy traditional-living peoples.

Japanese patterns of disease fly in the face of Western conventional wisdom. For example, they suffer one-fifth of the US lung cancer rate in spite of consuming nearly fifty per cent more cigarettes than Americans. That they have no genetic protection is shown by emigrants to America who rapidly approach the cancer incidence of the American population.

Japanese children have uniformly high IQs and are industrious and fired with the will to succeed in school, both in Japan and the US. Their standards of education are the highest in the Western world*. But those of the younger generation who emulate the Americans and eat beef and milk are taller than their parents, and have crowded teeth with more Western rates of decay. How long

*A footnote for the sceptical. When the New York school system banned products with more than 10% sugar, preservatives or food colouring, academic performance went up by 15.7% over other school systems on an academic ranking scale. The standard deviation for each school system's annual change in this ranking was less than 1%, *which is to say that it's highly unlikely, statistically speaking, that this was a fluke* (S. Schoenthaler, 'Testing of Various Hypotheses as Explanations for the Gains in National Standardized Academic Test Scores in the 1978-83 New York City Nutrition Policy Modification Project', *Int. J. Biosocial Research*, (1986), 8(2):196-203)

before they emulate the American incidence of broken homes, drug addiction and birth defects?*

## *What Can We Do?*

Whatever our state of health, Sinclair's high ratio of essential to non-essential oils in the diet will improve or preserve it. Those of us most at risk because of the Pottenger effect, illness or for whatever reason can return our essential fatty acid patterns towards that of health with supplementation.

Above all, we should protect those who are pregnant. We in the West have suffered generations of inadequate nutrition. We are, like Pottenger's cats, less than we could be. Through no fault of our own, we have lost some of our human qualities – but we can reverse this deterioration in our children.

* *In Health* magazine has estimated that by the year 2053, *half* of the American population will be in jail if the present rate of crime increase continues (September 1991).

# 5: Deranged Essential Fatty Acid Diseases

I'm a psychologist, not a doctor, but when I was diagnosed a diabetic, I felt that I had to try to solve the medical puzzle of surviving diabetes because the prognosis is generally so bad – up to a third off your life expectancy. Luckily for me, some far-sighted people have stepped beyond the bounds of conventional wisdom to study the solution, and when I looked, the evidence was there. Moreover, I found a new way of looking at other life-threatening diseases which gives hope for healing.

Drs Hugh Sinclair[1], David Horrobin[2], Charles Bates[3] and others have compiled an extraordinary list of diseases caused by unbalanced essential fatty acids. Here they are in rough order of the number of people they affect. Conditions given in ***bold italic*** have sections to themselves in this chapter.

***Ageing***
***Food Allergy***
Dental Caries (tooth decay)
***Cosmetic Changes*** (wrinkled skin, dandruff, brittle nails, etc.)
Depression, ***Irritability***
Viral Infections (Poliomyelitis, ***Chronic Fatigue Syndrome***, etc.)
***Overweight***
Atherosclerosis and the Thrombotic diseases:
  Atherosclerosis and Coronary ***Heart Disease***
  Cerebrovascular Disease (stroke, premature senility)

Pulmonary Embolism (a stroke in the lung)
Phlebitis (veins blocked by clots)
***Cancer*** of the Lung and Stomach, Leukaemia
***Rheumatoid Arthritis***
***Alcoholism***, Cirrhosis of the Liver
The Complications of ***Diabetes***
Atopic Eczema, Asthma, ***Hyperactivity in Children***, Cystic Fibrosis
Gallstones
Endometriosis
Peptic Ulcer
Nephrosis and Renal Stones
Pre-Eclampsia (high blood pressure in ***Pregnancy***)
***Acne***
Slipped Discs, ***Osteoporosis***
Appendicitis
Ulcerative Colitis, Irritable Bowel Syndrome, Diverticulosis
***Multiple Sclerosis***
Collagen diseases:
Ankylosing Spondylitis
Arteritis (inflammation of the arteries)
Systemic Lupus Erythematosus
Polyarthritis Nodosa
Rheumatic Fever
Crohn's Disease
Scleroderma (skin of face and hands hardens)
Hypercalcaemia of Infants (too much calcium in the blood)
Sjögren's Syndrome (low tears and saliva)
Sjögren-Larsson's Syndrome (scaly skin, retardation and spasticity at birth)
Schizophrenia

Most of these conditions worsen with age in the West, as one might expect since both fatty-tissue linoleic acid and the 'delicate first step' enzyme decline with age. However, traditional diets such as that of the Japanese preserve fatty-tissue LA, and consequently (I believe) Japanese cholesterol levels and blood pressure remain relatively stable with age and *the Japanese do not deteriorate with age as we do.*

This is the secret of preserving our looks, intelligence and vigour into old age. Now we can 'die young as late as possible!', as Dr Ashley-Montagu put it. Here are the answers that I looked for so desperately when I learned I had diabetes, and they turn out to be a generic solution for our peculiarly Western diseases!

Essential fatty acid therapy actually prevents some of these conditions. It halts deterioration in many, like Multiple Sclerosis, or even reverses it, as with diabetic complications. All probably respond to dietary improvements which raise Sinclair's ratio*. Those which stem from defective enzyme activity (whether congenital, from the Pottenger effect**, ageing or disease) are further helped with GLA from evening primrose oil and omega-3 derivatives from fish. But here's a surprise: many are made worse by certain foods, and, in some cases, *no amount of dietary improvement helps until the offending food or foods are removed from the diet* – see **Food Allergy, Food Addiction**, page 151.

So join me in this adventure. Let us see how to repair the balance of the EFAs in these diseases. This is the emerging paradigm, a shift in the world picture, as when James Lind found the cure for scurvy or Jonas Salk discovered his polio vaccine. Things will never be the same, and things can be better – but only if we grasp the nettle and understand for ourselves.

## *Acne*

In 1988, H.C. was a bright young red-haired woman with skin so riddled with acne that my wife nearly didn't hire her as a

*Epidemiologically, these diseases are more common wherever Sinclair's ratio of essential fatty acids to saturated fat plus trans fats is low. The UK diet has a ratio of about 0.2, and we suffer substantially. UK vegetarian diets have higher ratios, and the vegetarians among us suffer correspondingly less. In striking contrast, the diets of Japanese farmers and traditional Eskimos have ratios of 1 and 1.4 respectively, and they are virtually immune from the degenerative diseases which kill us, although they do have more high blood pressure, strokes and stomach cancer than we do (H.M. Sinclair, 'Essential Fatty Acids in Perspective', *Human Nutr. Clin. Nutr.*, 1984, 38C:245-260).

**The Pottenger Effect is the deterioration and atopy developing over several generations of poor diet.

personal assistant because it was literally difficult to look at her. Her father was an alcoholic, and her immediate family contained Scots, Irish and Scandinavian blood. She was anorexic as a teenager, and therefore probably zinc-deficient. My wife found her able and articulate for most of the month, but in her premenstrual week she'd burst into tears at the slightest provocation – in short, a perfect candidate for essential fatty acid therapy! Here is her story.

> 'In January of 1989, I started out on a daily programme of Borage Oil*, Vitamin A**, and *Optivite* PMT. At that time, I also made a change in my diet to include more seafood, and to eliminate processed sugars and oils, most dairy products and caffeinated beverages and sodas. For about seven years prior, I had been having trouble with acne which no antibiotic treatment seemed able to cure, and I had symptoms of Premenstrual Syndrome (achy back, weight gain, mood swings, irritability) since I was thirteen. The effects took about two weeks to manifest. My skin calmed down, and my temperament became more stable.
>
> 'At the end of March of 1989, my diet slipped and the acne began to reappear. I began supplementing with two tablespoons of devitaminized cod liver oil each day . . . I continued on this programme until November, at which time I cut back to half my original programme (6 *Optivite* and 5 Borage Oil capsules) and discontinued the cod liver oil.
>
> 'The results have been dramatic. My skin is virtually clear, and if symptoms of PMS occur, they are much less severe and are usually more directly related to external stresses . . . fringe benefits have included a six pound weight loss as well as an enormous boost in energy. I believe I have been better able to concentrate since I began using this programme.'

*Borage Oil contains GLA but evening primrose oil might have been more effective – see page 101.

**This was 'mycelized' vitamin A, tiny droplets suspended in water, and provided 100,000 IU per day. This kind of megadose should only be taken under medical supervision because of the risk of vitamin A toxicity.

I was amazed when I saw her again. Instead of a fiery red complexion with weeping acne, she had clear, milky-white skin with only traces of redness left in the middle of her cheeks. Her confidence and disposition have improved to the extent that she's now achieving her ambition to become a writer, which is what she always wanted to do but never believed she could.

## *Ageing*

> ***Everyone faces at all times two fateful possibilities: one is to grow older, the other not.***

In the West, ageing people have rising cholesterol levels*, blood pressure, declining kidney and heart function and increasing auto-immunity**, which shows up in diseases like rheumatoid arthritis. In marked contrast, populations existing on more unrefined, traditional diets have a profoundly lesser incidence of these degenerative conditions.

The enzyme needed for the 'delicate first step' of essential fatty acid metabolism declines with age, first in peripheral tissues and finally in the liver***. Multiplying the effect of this decline, levels of linoleic acid in body fat fall with age in Westerners (but not in Japanese men[4]). Accordingly, it is not surprising to discover that elderly Western men with heart disease have the characteristic pattern of EFA derivatives we saw on page 94 in Chapter 3[5], nor that elderly Japanese men are unlikely to have heart disease at all.

All this suggests that essential fatty acid replacement therapy will be helpful in the aged, and that some of the deterioration we now accept as inevitable may be postponed, slowed or even prevented. Examples include the thrombotic diseases such as heart attacks and strokes, rising blood pressure and cholesterol, rheumatoid arthritis and the premature senility caused by atherosclerosis.

*Only 13% of men and 10% of women between 50 and 64 have safe cholesterol levels (*The Times*, 15 June 1990)

**This age-related rise in auto-immunity is associated with lessened T-suppressor lymphocytes, possibly a consequence of falling PGE1 levels.

***The most prominent declining enzyme is the 'delicate first step' delta-6-desaturase enzyme.

There should be considerable improvements in appearance, since the deterioration in elderly skin is a clear indicator of the decline in the essential fatty acid metabolism in the liver.

Interestingly, one strategy shown to slow ageing and extend the lifespan of laboratory animals is a low-calorie diet, and there is some evidence that this is effective in humans*. Such diets have been seriously proposed for people[6]. That *caloric restriction increases the activity of the 'delicate first step' enzyme by up to three times* may be the explanation[7]. Support this fragile enzyme with the steps in Chapter 2!

# *Alcoholism*

To the Navajo people, whiskey is 'todilhil', the water of darkness.

I think that we accept alcohol's incredible destruction of our lives in road deaths and violence because we are literally so ill-nourished. Alcohol for many of us is self-medication for depression which leaves us even more ill-nourished, and ultimately helpless against its temptation. For others, genetically defenceless, it's an almost irresistible corrupting force.

## TWO DRINKS A DAY

Surprisingly, people who have two drinks a day live longer than teetotallers and much longer than heavier drinkers[8]**. Some believe that the small quantity of alcohol may raise low PGE1 levels by stimulating the release and conversion of DLGA, while

*For example, Louis Cornaro was a Venetian centenarian who lived from 1464 to 1566 and wrote *La Vita Sobria* towards the end of his life. He was convinced that his very restricted diet restored his health and was responsible for his remarkable longevity. Louis Cornaro, *The Art of Living Long*, William F. Butler, Milwaukee, 1905.

**That two drinks per day improves health is a Western statistic, and may only be true where diets have a low Sinclair's ratio (see footnote, page 115). Factors other than the PGE1-stimulating effect of alcohol may be at work. For example, copper deficiency can cause atherosclerosis, but rats drinking beer were protected while those drinking alcohol and water were not. Both groups were fed a low-copper diet, and the trace quantities of copper in the beer could not have protected them. The researchers theorized that something in the beer potentiated copper uptake ('Give That Rat A Bud', *Discover*, September 1990).

heavier drinking inhibits the 'delicate first step' enzyme and blocks the essential fatty acid metabolism of linoleic acid[9]. Consequently, heavy drinkers develop the characteristic disturbance of essential fatty acid derivatives seen on page 95.

Perhaps this explains why some people drink moderately for years before becoming heavy drinkers. Alcohol provides relief for their low mood by raising PGE1, but when their reserves of DGLA become exhausted, then heavier drinking is needed to stave off worsening PGE1-deficiency depression. *Two drinks a day may be, then, a dangerously unstable situation.*

But why is PGE1 low in the first place? Perhaps because of the Pottenger effect (page 94), northern coastal ancestry, trans fats, vitamin deficiency or simply too much fat. We put many obstacles in the way of our essential fatty acid metabolism. If this is the case, then *giving GLA as evening primrose oil might preserve DGLA levels and prevent alcoholism.* That evening primrose oil given to rats with alcohol *blocked the development of tolerance*[10] supports this reasoning*. It seems likely that the supplement preserved DGLA stores and prevented descent into rodent alcoholism.

## ABSTINENCE A MUST?

It is a tenet of Alcoholics Anonymous that 'wet ones'** must 'hit bottom' before their decision to stop drinking has a chance of success. Alcoholism is a disease of psychological denial, and alcoholics will incorporate anything that justifies continued intake – including evening primrose oil. Alcoholics Anonymous, the most successful alcoholic support network in existence, has only about a 30% success rate, but *offers no nutritional guidance whatsoever.*

However, Alcoholics Anonymous meetings are renowned for bottomless coffee urns and sugary snacks. It is most interesting that caffeine and sugar, like alcohol, inflame the gut and allow partially digested food molecules to pass into the bloodstream.

*However, giving EPO once alcoholism has developed sometimes actually increases consumption.

**In Alcoholics Anonymous, a problem drinker is called a 'wet one.'

Some believe that chemicals released when the immune system attacks these food molecules act like pain-killers in the brain[11]*, and that this may be a cause of addiction.

In the light of this, it makes sense that there seems to be a cross-addiction effect among these substances, and that avoiding all of them is often easier than avoiding any one of them. A practical suggestion for all who are trying to lower their intake of alcohol, caffeine or sugar is, therefore, to avoid all three. However, the theory also suggests that a more or less painful withdrawal period is likely when one stops, and I have seen evidence of this as well.

## The Genetic Connection

Some American Indian tribes have a very high incidence of alcoholism, suggestive of a genetic connection, and northern coastal peoples such as the Scots, Irish, Welsh, Scandinavians have the predisposition towards alcohol which was mentioned in Chapter 1.

Interestingly, Dr Charles Bates found that evening primrose oil alleviated fatigue and depression in more than 8 out of ten people who had 25% or more northern coastal ancestry, but helped only 3 out of ten who had other racial backgrounds. *Those who responded to EPO almost all reported depression during hangovers, while the non-responders didn't.* Dr Bates may have identified depression during hangovers as a marker for a genetically fragile essential fatty acid metabolism[12]**.

I take this to mean that alcoholism is a disturbed-EFA-derivative disease which people with fragile EFA metabolisms (whether from genes or diet) are more prone to. Evening primrose oil and the ***Food for Vitality*** programme will almost certainly help. However, my psychological training and experience in treating alcoholics

*All known addictive substances stimulate dopamine-sensitive fibres in the median forebrain bundle, and it has been shown that a component of the immune-system complement cascade behaves like dopamine in the hypothalamus.

**Dr Bates found that EPO disagreed with northern coastal fish-eating American Indians (probably because they share inactive D5D and D6D enzymes with the Eskimos and therefore need very little DGLA), but had positive effects in 'well over 90%' of others with a northern coastal background.

tells me that even with dietary improvement and supplementation, the 'denial' part of alcoholism is still likely to require treatment in the 10% of drinkers who drink 50% (!) of all alcohol consumed[13].

## Are We Doing The Right Thing?

In the UK, we maintain on very slim evidence that controlled drinking through education is possible for alcoholics. Cynics have suggested that this approach is much cheaper in terms of detoxification facilities and beds than the alternative approach of abstinence.

Whatever the merits of this debate, I suspect that those who abstain on will-power alone (so-called 'white-knuckle' alcoholics) have the most to gain from this book's dietary improvements, although all who use alcohol stand to benefit.

## Nick

Perhaps you have a Nick in your family. Nick is rather far along the primrose path to alcoholism, and I suspect it would take a full-scale intervention to get him to confront his dependence. Such confrontations are certainly not the province of diet books – but what if his dependence can be lessened with supplementation and dietary improvements?

## Help for Hangovers

Of immediate interest to drinkers is vitamin C and evening primrose oil's effect on hangovers. The consensus of numerous professional and amateur researchers is that taking vitamin C* and evening primrose oil capsules while drinking** greatly reduces distress the next day.

*500 mg of vitamin C per ounce of alcohol – vitamin C is known to speed the liver's clearance of alcohol from the bloodstream.

**Approximately one capsule per ounce of alcohol. O.E. wrote that she 'liked a glass of wine with dinner, but had to give it up because I felt dizzy at half a glass, and hungover the next morning if I drank any more. Since I started on 3 *Efamol* a day, I can enjoy a glass of wine without feeling sorry later!'

Beyond hangovers, alcohol withdrawal symptoms such as the pink elephants of Delirium Tremens are considerably lessened by evening primrose oil supplementation, *which also speeds liver and brain recovery*[14].

## Cancer

In 1900, cancer killed one in thirty. Today, it kills about one in five, *a 600% increase*. Deaths from cancer are higher than at any time in the history of the human race.

Sinclair's ratio* of essential fatty acids to saturated fats plus trans fats has barely changed from 0.2 since 1909, but fat consumption has gone up about 25%[15]. We know that cancer incidence goes up with fat consumption** – but if this is true, how is it that traditional-living Eskimos eat the same amount of fat as we do, and cancer is unknown amongst them? Cancer is also very low in Japanese people***. For example, the Japanese smoke a great deal more than we do, yet their lung cancer rate is one fifth of ours. There is one common factor between these populations – *Eskimos and traditional-living Japanese are exposed to negligible trans fats in food.*

Did the 1911 introduction of hydrogenation so change the *character* of today's fats as to cause this epidemic of cancer? Dr Johanna Budwig of Freudenstadt, West Germany****, thinks it likely.

### HUMAN AERIALS?

Dr Budwig believes that we can absorb energy from the sun's rays because our cell membranes are made up of essential-fatty-acid-

*Sinclair's ratio is discussed on page 115.

**In mice, a study showed that mouse offspring were *five times more likely to get cancer if their mother had been fed a diet rich in fat during pregnancy* (J. Raloff, 'Mom's Fatty Diet May Induce Child's Cancer', *Science News*, 1990, 137(1):5). Another study suggests that women detected in screening to be at risk from breast cancer were half as likely to develop cancer if they switched to a low-fat diet ('Breast Cancer: Low-fat Finding', *Science News*, 1988, 134(19):302).

***Other than gastric cancer, thought to be related to high salt consumption.

****Dr Johanna Budwig, Hegelstrasse 3, 7290 Freudenstadt-Dietersweiler, Germany. Tel. (0744) 5851

containing lipoproteins* whose electrons resonate at just the right frequency**. According to her, this energy is the spark which initiates and guides the Krebs cycle, the chemical process by which we obtain energy from the food that we eat[16]***. Stated like this, her theory calls to mind little green men with TV aerials on their heads. However, it may not be as batty as it seems.

## Warburg's Anaerobic Cancer Cells

Nobel Laureate Otto Warburg is famous for his observation that cancer cells rely heavily on anaerobic metabolism****. In plain English, this means the Kreb's cycles of cancer cells are defective, and the oxidation of glucose stops at lactic acid, releasing only 10% of the energy possible from the full reaction. Consequently, terminal cancer patients suffer from cachexia, in which tumours gobble up huge quantities of glucose and release lactic acid which the liver must laboriously turn back into glucose. The patient wastes away because of the inefficiency.

## A Seminal Observation

Warburg saw that within 24 hours after fatty-acid-containing sea urchin eggs were fertilized with protein-containing spermatozoa,

*These lipoproteins consist of essential fatty acids combined with sulphur-containing amino acids like cysteine and methionine. Interestingly, it is these very amino acids which cooking renders most resistant to digestion (D. Pieniazek et al., 'Methionine and cysteine in the formation of bonds resistant to the action of proteolytic enzymes in heated casein', *Br. J. Nutr.*, 1975, 34:163-173)

**A little quantum-physics background may help clarify this. Two photons of light form each electron which orbits the nuclei of atoms. These electrons can absorb further photons and become more energetic, or they can give out photons of light and fall to a less energetic orbit. Thus, light can excite matter and transfer energy to it, just as when the sun warms a stone. Budwig believes our enzymes can use this energy to catalyze the energy-producing reactions of the Krebs cycle.

***Udo Erasmus's *Fats and Oils* (Alive Books, Vancouver, 1986) lays out Johanna Budwig's programme in detail.

****Aerobic respiration powers cells with the sun's energy stored in the chemical bonds of fatty acids and sugars, put there by photosynthesis in plants. Anaerobic respiration powered life before there was oxygen in the atmosphere. Has the cancer cell fallen back on this incredibly ancient process because conditions in the body can no longer support aerobic respiration?

oxygen consumption increased by an amazing 2200%. In 1926, he therefore tried to rekindle the aerobic metabolism of cancer cells by adding fatty acids. He failed because he used butyric acid, a saturate found in butter which lacks unsaturated bonds*.

## Budwig Validates Warburg

In the forties, Johanna Budwig was a physicist consulting in West Germany for the Federal Institute of Fat Research, the government's adviser on nutritional fats and health. Because previous investigators were so hampered by the lack of laboratory techniques for analyzing mixtures of fats, the first task she set herself was to develop 'determinative lipid paper chromatography', a precise method for separating and measuring blood fats which is now used for blood analysis all over the world[17].

Budwig repeated Warburg's experiment in 1951, but she gave the cancer cells a tiny quantity of linoleic acid instead of butyric acid, and her observation that oxygen consumption increased many times over showed that she had succeeded where Warburg had failed. She had *rehabilitated the cancer cells' aerobic metabolism and made normal cells of them once more***.

Intrigued, she saw that a chromatograph blood fraction which in healthy patients fluoresced blue was yellow-green in blood from cancer patients and moved more slowly. When she added a tiny quantity of linoleic acid, the fraction turned red and moved faster

*This choice is all the more surprising because Meyerhof noticed in 1920 that adding essential-fatty-acid-rich flaxseed oil to frog muscle increased oxygen consumption a thousand-fold (O. Meyerhof, Naturwissenschaft, Pflugers Archiv., (1920) 8:696).

**It seems both EFAs and sulphur-containing amino acids are together necessary for health. More active tissues contain more of both. Animals are more sensitive to toxins if deprived of either, and starving animals die faster if fed either than those deprived of all food. In Italy (where tissue levels of the EFAs are high), but not in the USA (where tissue EFA levels are lower), sulphur-containing amino acids ameliorate liver and skin diseases, eclampsia in pregnancy and speed recovery from anaesthesia, possibly because anaesthetics are quite toxic. Udo Erasmus, *Fats and Oils*, Alive Books, Vancouver, Canada, 1986.

– haemoglobin!* Working backwards, she learned that the yellow-green proto-haemoglobin was 'cytochrome-c', a member of the chain of respiratory enzymes essential for aerobic metabolism and *the exact point at which respiration is blocked in cancer cells***.

Then she discovered 'polymerized fats of marine origin' in soft tumours[18]. Interestingly, an American analysis also implicated trans fat consumption and cancer of the breast, colon and bowel occurring ten years later***. Recognizing that the soft-tumour fats must come from whale-oil margarine, she prepared to warn the world of the danger she had discovered.

## The Margarine Connection

Unfortunately, she was working for a man who held patents on the hydrogenation process! Out of a job, and with the edible-oil interests against her, she lost the credibility necessary to publish her research in scientific literature****.

She set up as a nutritional practitioner in the country and

*Clinically, the yellow-green material is said to disappear from cancer patients blood in about three months on the Budwig programme.

**Cancer patients are usually anaemic, and Budwig interpreted her result to mean that they could no longer make haemoglobin because of an essential fatty acid deficiency. Such a deficiency would also account for cancer cells' frequently having two sets of genes, called polyploidy, for the next step in reproduction is cell-membrane manufacture which would require essential fatty acids.

***'The significant positive correlation for vegetable fat [with cancer] could not always be explained by the effects of the total unsaturated components; individual unsaturated components, such as oleic or linoleic acids; or the saturated component; but could be explained by the trans fatty acid component.' The oils used in studies showing polyunsaturated oils cause cancer in rats usually contain up to 17% trans fat, which casts doubt on whether high polyunsaturates or the trans fats cause the cancer (M. Enig et al., 'Dietary Fat and Cancer Trends – a Critique', *Federation Proceedings*, 1978, 37:2215-2220).

****Are we to believe that these forces have kept the news from our shores these forty years? If there is such a conspiracy of silence, then the hydrogenation process must be profitable indeed! Of course, Johanna Budwig's books are all in high German, and she has been pre-occupied in litigation with the medical establishment for upwards of thirty years. Perhaps the real surprise is that she has survived to well over 80 years of age, with her practice intact, her theories unrefuted and a steady stream of legal victories behind her.

prepared to perform the clinical experiment suggested by her laboratory results; namely, to cure cancer with diet. Reasoning that the essential fatty acids combine with sulphur-containing amino acids to form the lipoproteins in skin, cell membranes and all membranes within the cell*, she gave her patients flaxseed (linseed) oil combined with fermented unpasteurized skimmed milk ('kwark', a good source of sulphur-containing amino acids) in large quantities**, accompanied by carrots (for beta-carotene), fresh greens (vitamin C), whole grains and aromatic herbs such as cinnamon and anise***. By 1956, she was sure that she had a programme which cured cancer.

## SURPRISE, SURPRISE

She quickly found that a host of diseases such as diabetes, atherosclerosis, liver disease, muscular dystrophy, skin problems, arthritis and even diseases of the secretions (such as Sjögren's Syndrome in which tears and saliva decline) responded. With the passage of time, her list has come to look very like that at the beginning of this chapter.

In a further experiment, she tested her idea that man needs energy from the sun to 'kick start' the Krebs cycle. Using quantum physics, she calculated that the resonant frequency of the lipoprotein pi-electrons**** was 6900 angstroms, in the red part of

*Including the mitochondria, the tiny cellular power stations in which glucose and fats are oxidized for energy to power the cell, and which fail to perform in cancer.

**To make Johanna Budwig's 'oil-protein combination', add 400 grams of skim-milk cottage cheese (which neatly replaces kwark) to 250 grams of flaxseed oil. Add sufficient milk (about 25 grams) to blend until the oil is no longer visible. During cancer treatment, 250 or more grams of flax oil may be taken a day in this combination.

***Aromatic herbs such as fennel, coriander, thyme, lemon peel, vanilla, cacao and cloves apparently contain electron bonds similar to those in the essential fatty acids.

****Pi-electrons are the pairs of electrons which form the 'cis- methylene-interrupted pi- double bonds' in the essential fatty acids. Such bonds are bent, so that an essential fatty acid with two or three bonds is bent into a J or U. In the crook of the J or U, a cloud of pi-electrons remain loosely associated with the atoms they belong to, providing a conductive path for electrons in oxidative respiration, and, according to Budwig, an 'aerial' for receiving energy from the sun.

the visible spectrum. She bombarded patients with red light from a ruby laser – and, according to her, they got better faster! In a 1967 Stuttgart radio interview she said that 90% of even advanced cancers in whom radiation and surgery had failed responded to her methods.

She believes that cancer is incurable unless the link between light and lipoproteins is taken into account – but if we are well-nourished, the cancer cell is weak and vulnerable. To her, cancer-inducers are simply 'electron robbers', anything which prevents light from activating the cancer cells' Kreb's cycles. Those who lapsed from her diet and took margarine, butter, foods with animal fats or nitrate preservatives, chemotherapy drugs or even pain killers destroyed their lipoprotein pathways, diminishing their oxygen metabolism and inviting cancer to return.

Had I not discovered for myself how nutritional solutions to disease are greeted by such thunderous indifference and the amazing power of vested interests to influence research, I would probably regard the foregoing as the ravings of a nutritional lunatic*. Knowing what I do, however, I'd take long odds that Johanna Budwig has done what the cancer establishment has been trying to do for years – discover the cure for cancer.

## DR MAX GERSON, UNSUNG HERO

Much research corroborates aspects of her ideas. The great American clinician Dr Max Gerson[19], who spent forty years painstakingly experimenting with different foods until he produced a diet which cures cancer in many cases**, wrote to his

*Johanna Budwig's work remains unrefuted, although it can be tested with simple experiments. However, if the edible-oil interests are as powerful and as dangerous as has been suggested, then perhaps her colleagues' studied failure to acknowledge her work may have been intended to save her life.

**For example, Gerson found *by observation of human cancer patients* that certain vitamins (folic acid, A, E, $B_6$) and minerals (sodium, calcium, magnesium) actually accelerate the spread of cancer, although C, $B_3$, $B_{12}$, potassium and iodine could be given without danger. *This information is life-saving and unobtainable elsewhere.* Max Gerson, *A Cancer Therapy*, Totality Books, Del Mar CA, 1977, available from the Gerson Institute, 5012 Central Avenue #E, Bonita, CA 92002. Tel. (619) 267-1150.

friend Albert Schweitzer that he had 'succeeded in stimulating the fat metabolism without bringing the malignant cells back to life . . . [with] linseed oil. According to Johanna Budwig . . . [linseed oil] stimulates the tissues [which] comprise the defence and healing systems of the human body.'[20]

When I visited the Gerson clinic in Mexico, I met recovering cancer patients who had been sent home to die by their doctors. I learned that most burned or had allergic reactions in the sun when they arrived, but positively enjoyed being in the sun* after a little while on the Gerson programme, which includes flaxseed oil**. *When these cancer patients were given the dietary raw materials to repair the structural lipoproteins in skin, their natural capacity to withstand and even enjoy sunlight was restored, as Dr Budwig's theory suggested it would be.*

Should they prevail, I hope Drs Budwig and Gerson's incredible contributions will not be treated according to Sir James Mackenzie's aphorism:

> There are three stages in the history of every medical discovery. When it is first announced, people say that it is not true. Then, a little later, when its truth has been borne in upon them so it can no longer be denied, they say it is not important. After that, if its importance becomes sufficiently obvious, they say that, anyhow, it is not new!

*In Mexico, the midday sun can fry eggs. Sunlight is safer in the morning and evening when it is filtered through more of the atmosphere.

**Certainly, there is a strong literature attesting to the sun's beneficial health effects – see J. Ott, *Health and Light*, Pocket Books, NY, 1973 or Z. Kyme, *Sunlight*, WHP, Penryn, California, 1980. If we need both EFAs and sulphur-containing amino acids to withstand the sun, then the huge rise in skin cancer in the USA may be associated with their increased vegetable oil consumption. For example, in 1930, the risk of developing malignant melanoma was 1 in 1500. Doubling in the US just since 1980, and rising at a similar rate in 16 other nations, it is now 1 in 150 (*Science News*, 1988, 134(25):396). While the hole in the ozone layer and the increased popularity of sunbathing must contribute, the implication of Budwig's theory is that too much of our oil is in the trans form and there is too little available sulphur-containing protein in our diets.

## Essential Fatty Acids in Human Cancer Treatment?

In fact, essential fatty acids have already been used in human cancer therapy. Terminal cancer patients in South Africa were treated with up to 30 capsules of *Efamol* per day[21]. Of the 21 patients who began the study, all survived at least twice as long as expected. One was killed in a car accident with no evidence of cancer, one died of pneumonia and four were still improving at the time of writing.

It is well known that cultured cancer cells are without the 'delicate first step' of normal essential fatty acid metabolism[22], and current research reveals that, as might be expected, certain EFAs* kill cancer cells in the laboratory[23]. Similar experiments almost all suppose the position that the EFAs have strong anti-cancer activity[24].

Even the normally staid journal *Nutrition and Cancer* has published research suggesting that EFAs have a role in cancer therapy[25]. Finding that linoleic and arachidonic acids were responsible for the natural anti-tumour activity of the small intestine, researchers verified that these fatty acids killed leukaemic mouse white cells in test tubes without damaging normal cells. A single injection containing linoleic acid saved 40% of mice infected with a cancer which killed the entire control group**.

## Raw Foods

The cornerstone of Dr Max Gerson's cancer therapy consists of a diet of raw vegetables, juiced or eaten whole. Modern science first thought that their beta-carotene content was protective, but now believes that there are dozens of interacting protective compounds and that the best protection is therefore to eat a wide variety[26].

Why raw? Because all the studies I've run across which consider

*Especially those with three and four double bonds.
**The cancers were Ehrlich ascites tumours.

the form in which the vegetables are eaten have *demonstrated that raw vegetables are a great deal more protective*[27].

Another benefit from raw foods involves the enzyme inhibitors which prevent beans, nuts and seeds from sprouting until the time is right. These inhibitors also defend against insect pests by preventing their digestive enzymes from working, so it was thought that they were highly undesirable for human consumption.

However, it's been found that small amounts of enzyme inhibitors not only blocked development of cancerous cells but actually *transformed them back into normal cells*. This amazing result suggests that you will benefit if you eat your apple cores, for there are enzyme inhibitors in the apple seeds[28].

## VITAMIN C IN CANCER TREATMENT

Drs Linus Pauling and Ewan Cameron gave 10 grams of vitamin C per day to terminal cancer patients and found that their survival time increased from an average of 50 days in the control group to 150 days for the vitamin C group[29]. A Japanese trial had a closely similar result[30]. The untreated control group were all dead after 174 days, while 18 of the 54-strong vitamin C group lasted for an average of 483 days, and six were still alive when the trial ended after 866 days.

## SABOTAGED RESEARCH?

However, two Mayo Clinic studies which were published in the prestigious *New England Journal of Medicine* claimed to show that vitamin C is worthless in cancer treatment. When I read them, I was deeply shocked to discover that both studies were booby-trapped! It was clear on careful reading that the studies were *designed* to prove vitamin C didn't work, while appearing to be open-minded and impartial*.

In the first study, 52 of the 60 vitamin C patients had received

*Could it be a mistake? Such incompetence is unlikely because the Mayo Clinic is world-famous for its conservative, rock-solid study designs. It's really very puzzling.

chemotherapy[31]. However, chemotherapy damages the immune system, which Pauling believes is boosted by vitamin C*. In other words, chemotherapy patients would be *expected to respond poorly* to vitamin C. Interestingly, the vitamin C group actually survived one third longer than the control group, *so the results actually supported Pauling's position that vitamin C is a palliative for cancer*!

In the second study, the vitamin C was stopped as soon as 'there was marked evidence of the progression of malignant disease', which happened after an average of 2.5 months in a two-to-three year study[32]. Stopping experimental treatments after, say, a 25% increase in tumour size is a standard protocol for testing toxic chemotherapy drugs, *but vitamin C has not been shown to be toxic in any quantity*. Unfortunately, stopping large doses of vitamin C suddenly is likely to cause 'acute induced scurvy' because vitamin C has a strong rebound effect[33]. This means that the more effective vitamin C is against cancer, the greater the danger to the patient of stopping vitamin C suddenly in this way, *and the faster the patient is likely to die.*

I suspect that we are seeing torpedo tracks here. In America, cancer is a multi-billion-dollar industry, and drug sales would go down if vitamin C was found to be effective against cancer. Some research committee probably sorted through thousands of funding applications until they found the ones with the right flaws to make vitamin C appear ineffective. Much research is underwritten by the very companies who have the most to lose from nutritional therapies.

Pauling and Cameron pointed out that their vitamin C patients 'entered a period of increased well-being and general clinical improvement. The benefits enjoyed by a majority of these patients included, in addition to increased well-being, relief from pain . . . with a fortunate few living on year after year in apparent good health.'[34] 'Their cachexia** and anorexia disappeared.'[35] So

*Researchers found that vitamin C-enhanced PGE1 production was responsible for killing cancer cells in their laboratory, so vitamin C may do its work by several pathways (N.S. Gardiner et al., 'Enhanced Prostaglandin Synthesis as a Mechanism for Inhibition of Melanoma Cell Growth by Ascorbic Acid', *Prostaglandins, Leukotrienes and Essential Fatty Acids*, 1988, 34:119-26)

**Rapid wasting.

whatever the merits of the survival issue, vitamin C is worth its trifling cost for the relief it provides.

## What Would I Do If I Got Cancer?

I would run, not walk, to the Gerson Clinic*, where I would undertake the full Gerson programme. I would probably take plenty of both evening primrose oil and vitamin C, and follow Johanna Budwig's** advice as well. I've always been a belt-and-braces man – but remember, prevention is easier than cure.

# *Chronic Fatigue Syndrome*

This pattern of continuing fever and weakness after recovery from a viral infection is often called Epstein-Barr Syndrome, but it actually often occurs after infection by other viruses such as herpes and measles. Symptoms of the chronic fatigue syndrome form some combination of mild fever, sore throat, painful lymph nodes, muscle pain, tiredness for more than 24 hours after even light exercise, headaches, joint pain without swelling and sleep disturbance. But the major, disabling characteristic is fatigue.

The cause is unknown, although of course there is the usual suggestion that it's psychosomatic. There is no known cure. However, *some viruses close down the 'delicate first step' of the essential fatty acid metabolism*, and some interesting research has followed up this clue.

For example, the seven of 20 subjects who had persistent fatigue after recovery from acute Epstein-Barr infection*** *also* had disturbed patterns of essential fatty acid derivatives[36]. Low LA together with low AA suggest a pattern similar to that of alcoholics****. The researchers speculated that lowered DHA (a

*Gerson Institute, PO Box 430, Bonita, CA 92002, USA. Tel. (619) 267-1150.

**Dr Johanna Budwig, Hegelstrasse 3, 7290 Freudenstadt-Dietersweiler, Germany. Tel. (0744) 5851

***Also known as infectious mononucleosis or glandular fever.

****Total serum fatty acids rather than phospholipids were measured in this study, but the proportions should remain comparable.

derivative of the omega-3 oil EPA) caused the chronic fatigue, since it is necessary for muscles to contract*.

Such a pattern should respond to the diet and supplements suggested herein, and another study has confirmed that this is so[37]. After fifteen weeks of 8 capsules of *Efamol Marine*** per day, 84% of the chronically fatigued subjects rated themselves improved, agreeing very closely with their doctor's independent assessment.

## WHAT HAPPENED TO ME

When I had Chronic Fatigue Syndrome, years before I'd ever heard of an essential fatty acid, my doctor told me that six months' bed rest might help, but little else could be done beyond taking white toast and lemonade when my stomach felt delicate.

Instead, I tried a treatment I'd read about in *Medical Hypotheses* by Dr Robert Cathcart, inventor of the artificial hip joint[38]. I took ten grams of vitamin C*** as mixed mineral ascorbates each hour until I reached 'bowel tolerance', meaning just before the onset of diarrhoea. A person in good health reaches this level after one dose of ten grams, but I took *140 grams* on the first day!

I reduced this almost unbelievable quantity by 15% to 120 grams the next day, and kept this level up for a week until my bowels once again told me that it was time for another 15% reduction. Steady reductions to 75 grams followed, and there I stayed for nearly three weeks. After that, my bowel tolerance dose dropped rapidly to a normal level of about 10 grams. Because of vitamin C's strong rebound effect[39], I reduced slowly to the three grams I have taken daily since then. I was finally free of chronic fatigue which had all but disabled me since my acute viral symptoms cleared, although I had some days of profound exhaustion during the treatment.

*Specifically, DHA is necessary for the slow phase of red-muscle contraction.

**Which contain 35 mg of GLA and 17 mg of EPA per capsule.

***Vitamin C as mixed mineral ascorbates is much easier to take than plain ascorbic acid, and also replenishes potassium, magnesium and calcium lost to diarrhoea. Available as 'Buffered Vitamin C Powder' in 240 gram bottles from Nutricology, 400 Preda Street, San Leandro, CA 94577-0489. Tel. (415) 639-4572

Cathcart believes that vitamin C operates as a 'non-rate-limited antioxidant', allowing a stronger immune response by fully arming white cells so that they can use their 'respiratory bursts' of free radicals to kill intruders and infected cells. Interestingly, Cathcart has tabulated the different bowel tolerance levels he found in his patients who had various diseases:

| Cathcart's Bowel Tolerance Vitamin C Doses* | |
|---|---|
| Normal | 4 to 15 |
| Exercise, anxiety, mild stress | 15 to 25 |
| Food allergy | ½ to 50 |
| Hay fever, asthma | 15 to 50 |
| Burn, injury, surgery | 25 to 50 |
| Cancer, Rheumatoid Arthritis | 15 to 100 |
| Cold | 30 to 100 |
| Flu | 100 to 150 |
| Bacterial infections | 30 to 200+ |
| Epstein-Barr, viral pneumonia | 150 to 200+ |

However, neither Cathcart's immune-stimulating effect nor vitamin C's well-known anti-viral action could have contributed to my recovery because my antibodies against the Epstein-Barr virus had returned to normal before I started taking it. I think that the virus knocked out my essential fatty acid enzymes, and the massive excess of vitamin C stimulated whatever remained of my 'delicate first step' enzyme between LA and GLA, which needs vitamin C to work.

Whatever the mechanism, I am quite certain that Dr Cathcart's protocol does work, for both my sister, who had chronic fatigue for nine months, and A.P., a 54-year-old woman who'd had it for *four years* (and who'd tried every remedy she could find), responded as I did**. She wrote:

> 'Each day continues to be a miracle. I wake up alert (usually about 6 a.m.), keep going all day on the days I need to, come

*In grams per day. Compare this list with that in the footnote on page 155, which indicates what happens to vitamin C in some diseases.

**Note that all three of us abstained from alcohol completely to avoid liver damage while we were ill.

home and get dinner, and even sometimes do light reading or watch a movie in the evenings. On days when I don't start so early, or when I get a short nap in the afternoon, I can keep going till midnight or so without any strain. In other words, I'm really back where I was before I got this wretched illness! . . . I don't push myself the way I once did, but that's because I've discovered that I can do most of the things I really want to, and get more satisfaction from them, if I don't rush at them in the headlong way I used to do.'

There is further material on vitamin C on page 155. For more on vitamin C, see Linus Pauling's *How To Live Longer And Feel Better* (W.H. Freeman and Company, New York, 1986), and, if you can find it, *The Healing Factor* by Irwin Stone (Grossett and Dunlap, New York, 1972).

## Cosmetic Changes

Our skin, hair and nails betray our age and state of health. We spend a fortune on products and services which promise to improve them. The good news is that this book's programme restores all three to a healthier, more youthful state.

Signs of disturbed essential fatty acid levels can include:

- Acne
- Blackheads
- Brittle Nails*
- Cracked Fingertips
- Dandruff
- Dry Skin
- Dry, Brittle Hair
- Easy Sunburn
- Light Sensitivity
- Moist Palms**

*R.S. wrote 'My fingernails and toenails are definitely much stronger and healthier since I started *Efamol* and *Optivite*.'

**If accompanied by both thirst and strong urine, moist palms may mean a breakdown of the skin's capacity to contain moisture, caused by a functional EFA shortage. This is sometimes seen in hyperactive children.

- Oily Nose with Dry Cheeks
- Pimples
- Poor Vision in Darkness
- Rough Skin
- Slow-Growing Hair, Nails
- Thin Hair
- White Spots on Nails (also associated with low zinc)

The changes which take place in skin with age include thinning, wrinkling, age spots and sagging. *I've seen all these respond positively to this book's programme.* For example, blackheads were the bane of my adolescence, and I could only keep them under control with constant vigilance. They disappeared along with my oily nose problem for the first time in my life when I replaced fats with flaxseed (linseed) oil in my diet.

### BREAST SIZE

A welcome side-effect for some women who used evening primrose oil to combat PMS was an increase in cup size, without weight gain anywhere else. The cause is unknown, and the effect takes a minimum of six months to become noticeable[40].

## *Diabetes*

There are two kinds of diabetes. Young people get insulin-dependent diabetes when their pancreases stop making enough insulin, while older people get non-insulin-dependent diabetes which is caused by 'insulin resistance' preventing the body from using available insulin. Anyone who survives to 70 has a one-in-five chance of getting non-insulin-dependent diabetes. About a million Britons have diabetes, and, amazingly, about half of the non-insulin-dependent diabetics don't know they have it!* These people are at very high risk of the complications of diabetes, of which more later.

Left untreated, both kinds of diabetics get high blood-sugar

*About 60,000 new cases are detected in Britain each year, of which about 18,000 are children. *Another 20,000 new cases probably go undetected.*

which causes thirst and frequent urination (diabetes means 'siphon' or 'fountain') as the body tries to get rid of the excess blood sugar through the kidneys. Mineral depletion from all the urine production can cause muscle cramps, and glucose build-up in the eye blurs the vision. There may also be hunger with unexpected weight loss, slow-healing cuts, pins and needles and weakness. I first realized that something was wrong with me when I got muscle cramps, although I had no idea that it might be diabetes. The cluster of symptoms indicates diabetes quite reliably, and if more people knew of it, perhaps there would be fewer undiagnosed cases.

If these signs are ignored, insulin-dependent diabetics especially may get ketoacidosis, which occurs when acid by-products of protein and fat digestion upset the alkaline balance of the blood. There is a marked 'pear-drops' odour to the breath, tremendous thirst, dryness of the mouth and nausea. Untreated, ketoacidosis can progress to coma and death.

Oddly enough, insulin-dependent diabetes is more common in colder climates in the industrialized nations*, but traditional-living Eskimos are virtually immune. Taken with the fact that Japanese children have the lowest incidence in the West (1.7/100,000), this seems to indicate that *traditional diets rich in essential fatty acids protect against diabetes.*

## THE COMPLICATIONS OF DIABETES

Most diabetics eventually get complications thought to be caused by high blood-sugar, including blindness, heart disease, kidney failure, nerve damage or even gangrene. About 20,000 people a year die prematurely of diabetes-related illness in Britain.

The best strategy for minimizing diabetic complications is to keep the blood-sugar as near normal as possible with exercise, a blood-sugar monitoring programme using a portable meter with

*The incidence of insulin-dependent diabetes among children is 9.4/100,000 in sunny California and 20.8/100,000 in Vermont, where it gets quite nippy. This may have to do with the higher incidence of viral infections in colder climes, since insulin-dependent diabetes seems to be associated with such infections.

blood from a finger prick, a prescribed diet, weight loss if necessary and sugar-lowering pills or injections of insulin. Urine tests for glucose with reagent sticks are easy to perform, and can verify blood-sugar control.

Measuring Glycosolated Haemoglobin (HA1c), which is the amount of haemoglobin which has reacted with glucose (blood-sugar) in the bloodstream gives an indication of how good blood-sugar control has been over the preceding few months. High HA1c can predict, for example, the development of diabetic retinopathy* – in one study, 44% of those with high HA1c had severe retinopathy compared with only 2.9% of those with low values[41]. *Keeping HA1c as close to normal as possible is thought to be the key to minimizing the risk of complications.*

Paradoxically, such 'good control' of blood-sugar actually results in *more* episodes of low blood-sugar, or hypoglycaemia**. This is because what we mean by 'good control' doesn't come close to the exquisite regulation provided by a working pancreas. The extra sugar-lowering pills or insulin injections required to keep the blood sugar nearer the normal range increases the risk of inadvertent overdose and hypoglycaemia.

This, and the extra inconvenience of testing, means that 'good control' is not widely used. Less than 5% of diabetics self-test their blood-sugar and *two-thirds* of all diabetics do no testing whatsoever! Consequently half of all diabetics, on average, develop complications after seventeen years***.

*In diabetic retinopathy, fragile capillaries bleed into the eye and cause a progressive failure of vision. Nearly one quarter of all people with diabetes experience some visual impairment.

**Sudden implementation of the suggestions in this section practically guarantees hypoglycaemic episodes, so caution is advised! Don't make any changes in your diabetes-control regimen without consulting your doctor. The man who treats himself has a fool for a patient, etc.

***The last time anybody looked closely (circa 1956), the death rate for diabetic doctors was 35% *higher* than that of the general public (F.Dickinson et al., 'Physician Mortality, 1949-1951', *JAMA*, 1956, 162:1462-1468). Wags have suggested this was because of better compliance with their diabetologists' instructions (which included a *high-fat* diet at that time!), but it does suggest that an MD degree confers no survival advantage in this condition.

## HYPOGLYCAEMIA AND INSULIN REACTIONS

Hypoglycaemia means episodes of low blood-sugar caused by too much injected insulin or too many blood-sugar-lowering pills. From the diabetic's point of view, insight seems to drain away. Since self-awareness is the first thing to go, it's actually very hard for the diabetic to recognize his or her own hypoglycaemia, which may cause symptoms as diverse as day-dreaming and irritability, although it may be obvious to everybody else that something strange is going on.

If nothing is done to raise the blood-sugar, the severe hypoglycaemia which follows may cause the person to slur words, appear drunk and eventually collapse. Low blood-sugar is deeply uncomfortable because, for one reason, it negates the effects of the endorphines which control how much psychological pain we feel*. Consequently, *diabetics often feel depressed and low after hypoglycaemic episodes.*

There are really two kinds of insulin-dependent diabetics, those who have had hypoglycaemia and those who will have it. It is therefore very important to warn everybody so they know what to do when it happens.

## DEALING WITH HYPOGLYCAEMIA

First and foremost, *anyone who takes insulin or blood-sugar-lowering pills should carry some form of sugar with them.* It is better to have it and not need it than to need it and not have it. I carry two packets of sugar in my wallet, and this practice saved me when I'd taken insulin but was prevented from getting home for supper by a traffic accident.

Next, *work out a strategy with your spouse and colleagues for dealing with insulin reactions.* Anything which has been rehearsed is much easier for people with low blood-sugar to grasp. Fruit juice, a sugar cube or any food which will quickly raise the blood-sugar is needed, but, because diabetics have been told so often

*Interestingly, insulin shock, like electroshock, used to be used as a treatment for depression.

that 'sugar is bad', we may refuse such offers. Eye-contact, a firm tone of voice and a pre-arranged signal (such as 'I think your blood-sugar is too low!') are therefore important.

When hypoglycaemia has caused unconsciousness, nothing can be given by mouth but an injection of glucagon (available by prescription) will tell the liver to mobilize its reserves of stored sugar and restore consciousness*. Glucagon comes as a powder which must be mixed with a liquid in a complicated procedure before the injection, so it is vital that this, too, is rehearsed with whoever may have to administer the injection.

Having a plan for dealing with hypoglycaemic episodes makes good control a more attainable goal, so now let us go back to the problem of achieving good control.

## Good Control With Less Hypoglycaemia

By eating properly, you can have better control with fewer hypoglycaemic episodes. Furthermore, *the **Food for Vitality** eating programme will itself lessen the severity of complications, even if blood-sugar control cannot be improved.*

## Reduce Glycosolated Haemoglobin with Antioxidants

Remember that the amount of Glycosolated Haemoglobin (HA1c) in the blood tells us how good blood-sugar control has been over the preceding few months. The reaction between blood sugar and haemoglobin involves free radicals[42]**, so taking free-radical-neutralizing antioxidants such as vitamin C

*Remember, ketoacidosis from *high* blood-sugar control can also cause unconsciousness, and more *insulin* is needed to bring the person out of this 'diabetic coma'. Distinguishing between hypoglycaemia and diabetic coma is a doctor's job because the wrong treatment (giving insulin to someone who's hypoglycaemic) could kill them.

**This gem is *really* obscure, coming as it does from research into the so-called Maillard reaction between sugars and amino acids (the basic building blocks of proteins) which creates the delicious smells of cooking.

(3 grams)*, vitamin E (800 IU) and beta-carotene (50,000 IU) should lower the amount of HA1c formed in the bloodstream. Other undesirable reactions should also abate, and *antioxidants should therefore lessen the risk of diabetic complications.*

## Lowering Insulin Resistance

Insulin resistance means that the body can't use insulin efficiently so the pancreas has to make more to get the job done, resulting in higher-than-normal insulin levels in the bloodstream**. It is a risk-factor for (and also a cause of) non-insulin-dependent diabetes, but it is widespread among 'normal' people who have the characteristic spare-tyre 'apple pattern' of overweight (as opposed to the heavy-hipped 'pear pattern'). Such 'love handles' are also highly visible risk factors for heart disease and breast cancer[43]***. Unfortunately, good blood-sugar control itself can actually *cause* insulin resistance**** and apple-pattern weight gain in insulin-dependent diabetics![44]

However, Dr Houtsmuller of Rotterdam showed that insulin-dependent diabetics maintained the same blood-glucose levels with less insulin on linoleic-acid-rich diets (using ordinary safflower oil), which shows that *EFAs reduce insulin resistance*[45].

Other factors which lower the blood sugar include magnesium,

*This massive amount of vitamin C reflects the fact that vitamin C transport is insulin-dependent and therefore defective in diabetics – a dose of two grams failed to inhibit platelet aggregation in diabetics, although the dose had a marked inhibiting effect in normal men (*Thrombosis Research*, 1979, 15(5/6):639-50). Of course, antioxidants have many other uses in a body under siege like that of a diabetic.

**Paradoxically, *both* types of diabetics have high levels of insulin in the bloodstream. 'Peripheral hyperinsulinism' occurs because, normally, most insulin is used in the liver as soon as it's made by the pancreas next door, so insulin-dependent diabetics must inject extra to get the right amount to the liver. In Type II diabetes, the pancreas often makes *too much* insulin because insulin resistance reduces its effectiveness.

***Apple-shaped people have twice pears' risk of developing non-insulin-dependent diabetes.

****Apparently, the body lowers the number of insulin receptors in the face of too much insulin, making insulin less effective.

vanadium* and the chromium-containing Glucose Tolerance Factor found in foods like liver. Some foods elevate the blood-sugar less than others, so eating foods with a low 'Glycaemic Index' helps. Certain spices have insulin-like actions and can themselves lower the blood-sugar. There is also exercise**, soluble fibre, reducing stress and decreasing dietary fat, and we will discuss these tactics in turn.

## MAGNESIUM

Magnesium appears to be powerfully protective for diabetics. Researchers at the University of California at Los Angeles found that non-insulin-dependent diabetics with high blood pressure had lower-than-normal magnesium levels within their red blood cells, and their blood pressures became normal after just six weeks on magnesium supplements[46]***.

Similarly, a study at Osaka University found low magnesium in the plasma and red blood cells of poorly controlled diabetics (magnesium in their urine was higher also), and *those with the lowest magnesium levels had the severest symptoms of retinopathy*[47]. As mentioned, diabetic retinopathy occurs when the capillaries in the retina deteriorate until there is bleeding into the eye and a progressive failure of vision. 'Photocoagulation' with laser light can stop the bleeding, but there is no medically accepted strategy which will decrease the fragility.

*Vanadium not only potentiates insulin's action but also has an insulin-like action in the body. A 'Science' paper (22 March, 1985) indicated that vanadium normalized blood glucose and preserved heart action in animals, which is encouraging because most diabetics die of heart failure. Normal dietary intakes are from 10-2,000 mcg, but the insulin-like pharmacological effect requires much higher doses – 14 mg of vanadium was used in one human study without toxicity (*Diabetes*, January, 1990). Vanadyl sulphate is marketed for its steroid-like action, and 4 mg is equivalent to 22.5 mg of vanadyl sulphate.

**Insulin resistance is higher in the morning, which is one reason why it is sensible to exercise early in the day.

***The average blood pressures of the study participants went from 157/96 to 128/77 on 260 milligrams of magnesium chloride per day for six weeks.

# Chromium And The Glucose Tolerance Factor

Most Western people are depleted of chromium, which, combined with vitamin $B_3$ and glutathione*, forms the Glucose Tolerance Factor which works with insulin and increases its effect. A supplement containing 200–600 mcg of GTF may improve glucose tolerance, lower cholesterol and triglyceride levels, decrease insulin needs and even stabilize 'brittle' diabetes** in chromium-deficient people of all ages. Food sources include liver, kidney, brewer's yeast, mushrooms and spices, especially black pepper.

Chromium levels decline with age in the West but remain stable in traditional-living populations, possibly because refined foods both contain less and also increase urinary losses by up to 300%. The abrupt decrease found in women after childbirth may perhaps explain the diabetes of pregnancy, a fairly common complication which chromium supplements might prevent. Giving chromium supplements to old people with insulin resistance frequently normalizes their glucose tolerance test curves[48].

Significantly, chromium usually cannot be found in the aortas of people who die of heart attack, but it is present in the aortas of accident victims. If chromium deficiency can cause insulin resistance, this could be one reason overweight is a risk factor for heart disease***.

*Glutathione is a protein made of cysteine, glutamic acid and glycine, and found in brewer's yeast. One of its functions is to reduce the oxidized form of vitamin C (dehydroascorbic acid) to vitamin C once more in red blood cells. Diabetics frequently have fairly high dehydroascorbic acid, either because vitamic C transport is insulin-dependent or possibly because of low glutathione (M. Werbach, *Nutritional Influences on Illness*, 3rd Line Press, Tarzana CA, 1987).

**'Brittle' diabetes means the blood sugar is all but uncontrollable, soaring and plunging without apparent cause. Food allergies, *over*-use of insulin and stress can cause it.

***High circulating insulin is apparently a risk factor for heart disease independent of obesity or cholesterol level ('Hidden Heart Hazards', *Science News*, 136(12):184-86), perhaps partly because it induces fat synthesis within the walls of blood vessels, contributing to plaque formation ('Insulin-Stimulated Lipogenesis in Arterial Tissue', *Lancet*, 28 September, 1968).

# BEANS AND RAW VEGETABLES – THE GLYCAEMIC INDEX

Raw vegetables have much less impact on the blood-sugar than cooked, so much so that some insulin-dependent diabetics are able to give up the needle on a carefully chosen, entirely raw diet[49]. Similarly, eating from the right-hand side of the Glycaemic Index* chart which follows can help. However, ice cream and too much fruit are to be avoided because of their respective high fat and sugar content[50]**.

## GLYCAEMIC INDEX OF COMMON FOODS[51]

The effect of a food on the blood-sugar as a percentage of the effect of table sugar. ***Raw foods are in italics.***

| Food | GI | Food | GI |
|---|---|---|---|
| Glucose | 160 | Spaghetti, white | 77 |
| Potatoes, baked | 157 | Carrots, cooked | 74 |
| Honey | 147 | ***Grapes*** | 72 |
| Corn Flakes | 138 | Spaghetti, wholemeal | 71 |
| Weetabix | 127 | Baked beans, tinned | 70 |
| Bread, white | 116 | Bread, whole-grain rye | 67 |
| Bread, brown | 115 | Beans, kidney | 63 |
| Shredded wheat | 113 | ***Apple*** | 62 |
| Rice, white | 112 | Ice cream | 60 |
| Raisins | 102 | Beans, butter | 60 |
| **Table Sugar** | 100 | Yoghurt | 60 |
| Porridge Oats | 99 | Milk | 57 |
| Rice, brown | 97 | ***Pear*** | 55 |
| Potatoes, new | 94 | Milk, skim | 53 |
| ***Banana*** | 92 | Beans, haricot | 52 |
| Yam | 86 | Lentils | 50 |
| Frozen peas | 86 | *Peach* | 47 |
| All-Bran | 85 | ***Grapefruit*** | 42 |
| Potatoes, sweet | 81 | ***Plum*** | 40 |
| Parsnips | 78 | ***Cherries*** | 37 |

Notes: Raw fruits eaten whole score low in spite of their high sugar content. Raisins, which contain glucose, score high – but why so much higher than the grapes from which they came? Probably because the high temperatures used to dry commercial raisins actually cook them. The more cooking, the higher the glycaemic index, so canned beans also come well above beans cooked at home. Similarly, raw carrots barely affect my blood sugar, but cooked carrots send it through the roof. White bread has the same index as brown, a consequence of the dishonest commercial practice of colouring white bread with caramel and calling it brown. Note that *wholegrain* bread scores much lower.

## HERBS AND SPICES

Several common herbs and spices make insulin work better. No less an authority than the United States Department of Agriculture found that either bay leaves, cinnamon and ground cloves or nutmeg actually *tripled* insulin's action in the laboratory[52], implying that you will need less insulin if you eat lots of these spices. Herbalists have prescribed juniper and cedar berries[53] and Golden Seal[54], while Canadian doctors have used the roots of the Devil's Club shrub[55]***. The B-complex vitamin biotin in

*The Glycaemic Index is the area beneath the glucose response curve as a percentage of the area produced by the same number of calories as glucose. Collier found that the glycaemic index can actually predict how much the blood-sugar will be affected by a particular mixture of foods (G.R. Collier et al., 'Prediction of the Glycaemic Response to Mixed Meals in Non-Insulin-Dependant Diabetic Subjects', *Am. J. Clin. Nutr.*, 1986, 44:349-352). Interestingly, acorns rank among the foods with the lowest glycaemic index ever recorded. Acorns were a staple among the Pima Indians of Southern Arizona before they adopted modern refined foods and developed the highest incidence of Type II diabetes (40%) of any population group known ('Seeds of Protection', *Science News*, 2 June, 1990, 137(22):350-1). I find them quite palatable.

**Sugar from any source, including that from supposedly healthful glasses of fruit juice, impairs the immune system for at least three hours (A. Sanchez et al., 'Role of Sugars in Human Neutrophilic Phagocytosis, *Am. J. Clin. Nutr.*, 1973, 26:1180-84), although the fibre in the whole fruit slows absorption and prevents this effect.

***I tried 'Devil's Club Compound' from Herb Pharm (Williams, OR 97544, USA) and it reduced my insulin requirement by about 20%. It was, however, considerably more expensive than insulin.

large quantities has an insulin-like action which lowers blood-sugar[56]*.

## Soluble Fibre

A high-fibre diet and supplements of soluble fibre such as psyllium husks (in *Metamucil*) or guar gum lessen the rise in blood-sugar after a meal, making good control easier to achieve. A 'grazing' eating pattern of snacks works much better than three square meals a day for the same reason.

## EFAs Against Diabetic Complications

Diabetic complications affect blood vessels and capillaries in delicate tissues so that, for example, heart attack risk may be six times higher in diabetics. The reason is not known for sure, but it seems to be a more rapid action of the same mechanism as in normal people. As with normal people, the strategy for minimizing this risk is to eat a diet containing large amounts of the essential fatty acids found in seed oils and cold-water fish, and little non-essential fat. Apparently, this both gives the body the materials it needs to repair the blood vessels and helps keep the blood flowing freely.

## Dr Houtsmuller's Research

In a five-year study, the aforementioned Dr Houtsmuller of Rotterdam showed that *complications (especially diabetic retinopathy) stopped progressing or actually diminished in fifty-one adult-onset diabetics who took 13% of their calories as linoleic acid*, the equivalent of a couple of ounces of vegetable

*The dose of biotin was 16 mg per day, hundreds of times the physiological requirement. Serum biotin levels reached 100 times pre-treatment levels, and blood-glucose fell significantly.

oil[57]*. Complications progressed in fifty diabetics who ate the amount usually found in the Rotterdam diet (about 4%).

*This is an astounding result because no treatment has ever had such success in halting or reversing complications* – yet, since it is a dietary approach, it has sparked less interest than it deserves. For example, a *New England Journal of Medicine* review article, 'Diabetic Retinopathy, A Synthesis of Perspectives'** made no mention of Dr Houtsmuller's findings (even though these appeared in 1980 and 1982) and concluded that good blood-sugar control was the most promising way to mitigate retinopathy.

Dr Houtsmuller's strategy of replacing non-essential fat with essential fat improves matters in two ways. Firstly, there are more essential fatty acids for the enzymes to work on, and, secondly, there are fewer non-essential fats competing for the enzymes. Women fared better than men in his studies, and as men appear to have a higher essential fatty acid requirement than women, this probably means that Houtsmuller's diet is still below the optimum protective level. However, there is a limit to how much vegetable oil you can eat, so by-passing the defective processing step by supplying GLA from evening primrose oil (with EPA and DHA from fish) clearly makes sense.

In clinical trials, *evening primrose oil has decreased diabetic neuropathy*[58] (see page 99), so we know that we are on the right track. Again, extraordinarily, this finds no mention in an authoritative *New England Journal of Medicine* analysis entitled 'Diabetic Autonomic Neuropathy'.[59] Nerve damage from

*Houtsmuller found a strong inverse correlation between progression of retinopathy and serum cholesterol-linoleate. The Glucose Tolerance Tests and responsiveness to insulin improved markedly in the females of the experimental group (who benefited much more than the men). Heart attacks occurred only in those with the lowest cholesterol-linoleate levels, less than 40%. Retinopathy progression ceased when serum cholesterol-linoleate was greater than 55%. *Remarkably, even those with constantly elevated blood-sugar* (*in whom you'd expect large amounts of Glycosolated Haemoglobin – see footnote, page 137*) *were protected!*

**T. Merimee, 'Diabetic Retinopathy, A Synthesis of Perspectives', *New England Journal of Medicine*, 5 April 1990, pp. 978-983

diabetic neuropathy can cause tingling, pain, loss of sensation, feelings of muscular weakness, impotence in men, high blood pressure, bladder disorders, tummy trouble and irregular heartbeats.

It is quite clear that medicine has little interest in mitigating neuropathy or retinopathy with dietary essential fatty acids. However, since these conditions can make life miserable and deprive one of eyesight, *I suggest most strongly that diabetics anticipate these problems and forestall them with essential fatty acid therapy.*

## Optivite, A Source Of The EFA Co-Nutrients

The nutrients which support the essential fatty acid metabolism are zinc, magnesium, $B_3$, $B_6$ and C, and diabetics seem more prone than most people to suffer from shortages. Interestingly, women with PMT have a defect in essential fatty acid processing similar to that of diabetics. Accordingly, I find three or four tablets of *Optivite*, a premenstrual tension supplement, supplies these nutrients in the appropriate proportions and seems to stabilize my diabetes.

## The Motivation Problem

There is much a diabetic can do if he or she is motivated. However, the medical literature is loaded with titles like: 'Diet Therapy for Diabetes: An Analysis of Failure'[60], and diabetics often just don't act in their own best interests. I suspect this is caused by low PGE1 levels (an inevitable consequence of the distorted essential fatty acid pattern in diabetes) which both depresses mood and heightens the addictive effects of a poor diet. Correcting such a pattern should renew optimism and provide more strength to resist temptation by lessening appetite.

## Fish Oil Supplements Don't Agree With Diabetics

For some unknown reason fish oils such as cod-liver oil or *MaxEPA** increase insulin resistance in diabetics, but eating cold-water fish has no such effect, and their oils both increase GLA's effectiveness and provide additional protection against heart attack. GLA is a precursor of PGE1, which boosts insulin's effectiveness, in addition to its other desirable properties.

The signal that these steps are having the desired effect is that cholesterol levels will drop well below 200 mg/dl, with a good ratio of cholesterol to HDL (see page 163). Your doctor will find this deeply satisfying, and you will know that you have made your old age possible.

## Stress Control

Anxiety interferes with diabetic control by raising the stress hormones[61], increasing both insulin resistance and glucose production in the liver, so diabetics who are prone to anxiety would do well to consider one of the newer antidepressants. Prozac, for example, is a prescription antidepressant with a strong anti-anxiety effect and few side-effects. Prozac frequently does much to stabilize frisky blood-glucose levels and may even reduce 'brittle' diabetes (page 143).

Alternatively, melatonin is emerging as a natural tranquillizer. A derivative of the neurotransmitter serotonin, melatonin is made by the pineal gland deep within the brain during the hours of darkness, and appears to synchronize the body's activities. In addition, it has prolonged the lives of mice by 20%[62], reduced intra-ocular pressure[63] (a risk-factor for glaucoma), ameliorated jet lag[64], negated the effects of stress and protected against cancer in animal experiments[65] and is even a part of a birth-control pill which, it is hoped, will lessen the risk of breast cancer[66]. Interestingly, the opioid antagonist naltrexone blocked these good effects[67], indicating that melatonin probably potentiates the effect of our natural painkillers, the endorphins.

*Trademark of Seven Seas Health Care Ltd., Hull.

This fascinating substance is at the cutting edge of research today, and may herald a new era of natural tranquillizers which work by enhancing the body's tactics for dealing with problems. The subjective effect of taking it* (as pineal gland extract) is a good night's sleep without any hangover although too much leaves one feeling detached from oneself and irritable. I have found that it calms down my blood-sugar when I'm under stress, so that I awake with normal instead of elevated blood-sugar.

Perhaps the best advice for diabetics is to take an interest in their own condition. *Since the EFAs and their co-nutrients are the only treatments ever shown to be effective against the lethal complications of diabetes, those who choose to remain oblivious risk premature and probably uncomfortable deaths*. After all, it's not the fellow in the white coat who's going to get the complications, and, as Samuel Johnson remarked in 1777, 'when a man knows he is to be hanged in a fortnight, it concentrates his mind wonderfully!'

I don't intend this as a reflection on the medical profession. I am no doctor-basher, quite the opposite in fact. Doctoring means tried and tested remedies based on a profoundly valuable, *tested* body of medical knowledge. There is no such conservatism in the 'alternative' therapy field, and, while I'd leave no stone unturned, I'd very much prefer to have a doctor as my primary care-giver. Most diabetes specialists are completely unaware of this material, but doctors aren't trained in nutrition and do not usually hold themselves out as dietary experts.

Thus, when a new paradigm (such as the essential fatty acids) emerges, we who have the most to gain must risk the new therapy on ourselves. Luckily, there are no known side-effects to this approach, so the experiment is virtually without risk!

## SMOKING

Diabetics smoke as much as the rest of the population, even though *smoking doubles the death rate of insulin-dependent diabetic women* – and diabetic women already have a risk of death *ten*

*Marketed as *Chronoset* and *Stressguard* by Nutricology, 400 Preda Street, PO Box 489, San Leandro, CA 94577, USA. Tel. (415) 639-4572

*times* higher than non-diabetics. For men, the six-times greater risk stemming from diabetes increases to ten times if they smoke[68].

## IMMUNITY

Before I got diabetes, I had a couple of colds each winter. I would also have several 24-hour bouts of bronchitis with high fever in summer. In other words, my immune system was not terribly effective.

After I got diabetes, I experienced the typical decline in immunity and was plagued with fungus infections of the skin, as often happens with diabetics.

Since developing the way of eating described in this book, I have been healthy and free of infections for periods of years at a time, longer than at any time in my life! For someone with an immune system supposedly compromised by diabetes, this is remarkable!* I hope that you may experience the same effect.

# *Food Allergy, Food Addiction*

Six or seven years ago, I read about a diabetic New Hampshire architect who switched to a macrobiotic diet after a relative recovered from diabetes in a Japanese prisoner-of-war camp. He wrote, 'My weight dropped from 200 to about 160. I stopped drinking alcohol too, which I really didn't think was possible. By the end of my second month on macrobiotics I was down to six units of insulin a day [from 26 units].'[69]

As a result, I switched to a macrobiotic diet in search of better diabetic control, and was amazed when I, too, lost interest in alcohol. However, I'd been on a similar, Pritikin-style diet composed of foods I was used to, *which had no effect on my taste for alcohol.* These diets were almost identical in terms of calories and nutrients and so forth, but differed in that *the macrobiotic*

*One theory of how insulin-dependent diabetes is caused involved just such a series of viral infections as I had, culminating in an unfortunate immune-system attack on the insulin-producing cells of the pancreas. I'm sure this is what happened to me. I think my greasy diet lowered PGE1 until my immune system was hyperactive but ineffective, like someone who's drunk too much coffee, and perhaps it took against my insulin-producing cells because they resembled the viruses I suffered from so often.

*diet was composed of unfamiliar foods* like beans, brown rice and soy products.

I drink almost nothing now, although I've long since dropped the macrobiotic diet because my insulin requirement hardly changed, and alcohol seems attractive only when circumstances prevent me from following my PGE1-supporting way of eating, as when travelling. I'm convinced that the *change* of diet removed foods to which I reacted badly, *and that this restored my essential fatty acid metabolism.*

All this sounds bizarre, even to me. It's the kind of thing one would dismiss out of hand because it 'doesn't make sense'. However, *doctors have noticed that withdrawing foods has had profound beneficial effects in any number of diseases* which would not respond to conventional treatment.

## Food Allergies In The Medical Press

Reports in reputable medical magazines such as the *Lancet* and the *British Medical Journal* link food allergies to heart attack[70]*, atopy and irritable bowel syndrome[71], canker sores[72]**, agoraphobia, stomach-ache with fast heartbeat, and nausea[73]***, migraine[74], anaemia with bronchitis[75], rheumatoid arthritis[76,77]****, diarrhoea, headache, confusion, lassitude,

*Mortality after heart attack was increased three-fold if antibodies to cow's milk or egg white were present. Interestingly, heart patients' coronary arteries were hypersensitive to and contained elevated stores of histamine and serotonin, and mast cells which synthesize them were increased in proportion to atheroma. Thus, food allergy could trigger vasospasm and heart attack, while magnesium, a natural mast cell release blocker, should be protective (S. Kalsner, *Science*, 1984, 223:1435-37). Even more interestingly, there's a direct, linear relationship between milk protein consumption and heart attack rates in 24 countries! (S. Seely, 'Diet and Coronary Heart Disease: A Survey of Mortality Rates and Food Consumption Statistics of 24 Countries', *Medical Hypotheses*, 1981, 7:907-918)

**Of 12 patients with prolonged and relentless periods of ulceration, there were two spontaneous remissions and 6 who responded to exclusion diets (3 gluten, 1 milk, 2 azo dyes such as tartrazine). Interestingly, 5 had salivary gland atrophy more usually associated with Sjögren's Syndrome.

***Six patients responded to the exclusion of a single food: agoraphobia (tea), headache (coffee), canker sores (raw potato), tummy ache and fast heartbeat (tea or alcohol), nausea (tea) and hypertension (caffeine).

****Seven patients' symptoms worsened on challenge with egg (3), wheat (2), potato (1), or beef (1).

blocked nose, backache or depression[78]*, ear infections[79]** and hypertension[80]. Even multiple sclerosis has apparently remitted after foods were withdrawn[81,82,83]. The foods involved included milk, eggs, wheat, tea, coffee, the yellow food dye tartrazine (E102), potato, beef, banana and chocolate.

Although food allergies are not widely accepted by the medical fraternity, can there be so much smoke without a fire? It all seems to suggest that over-use of common foods somehow exhausts our capacity to utilize them properly, and the bewildering variety of resulting symptoms hints that the *EFA-to-prostaglandin pathway is involved*.

## Conventional Wisdom

'Allergy' means an immediate allergic reaction, but 'food allergy' has come to mean almost any adverse reaction to food, whether immediate, disguised or deferred. One link with the EFAs seems to be through prostaglandin E1, since giving synthetic PGE1 (as the prescription drug Cytotec***, used to treat ulcers) with problem foods often lessens food allergy symptoms. PGE1 both curtails gastric acid secretion and stimulates gut-protecting mucus production.

I suspect that food allergy symptoms are often caused by PGE1-deficient 'leaky guts'****, which allow partially digested food

*Of 33 patients, symptoms cleared in 36% and improved in 45%. Only 7 patients submitted to an unpleasant procedure (naso-gastric tube) to verify their symptoms were due to milk products (2), egg (2), wheat, banana and chocolate.

**78% of children with chronic ear infections were found to be sensitive to foods, including milk, wheat, peanuts and maize, and the ear infections remitted when these foods were withdrawn.

***Searle Laboratories makes Cytotec, a long-acting analogue of PGE1, for treating ulcers. It inhibits both gastric histamine secretion, protects the GI tract from alcohol and bile-induced irritation and inhibits aspirin-induced faecal blood loss. The PGE1 inhibitors caffeine, aspirin, sugar and alcohol all inflame the gastric mucosa, and Cytotec appears to be powerfully protective against their effects (C.E. Bates, 'Racially Determined Abnormal Essential Fatty Acid[s]', *Medical Hypotheses*, 1988, 25:103-109).

****As a food-allergy specialist remarked, 'talking about the clinical implications of leaky bowel syndrome pretty much guarantees pariah dog status in the scientific and medical communities.' A proof-reader told me that the very idea was disgusting to normal people. Perhaps these reactions are among the reasons food allergy effects are so consistently denied.

particles into the bloodstream where they cause immediate immune responses via immunoglobulin E antibodies, or delayed reactions involving immunoglobulin G antibodies. *Sugar, alcohol, caffeine-containing drinks and aspirin*[84]* *all boost leakage by inflaming the gut mucosa*[85] *and worsen food allergies, which supports this concept (see page 119).*

## THE LINK TO EFAS

Psychologist Dr Charles Bates had a unique opportunity to explore food allergy. When he moved from a predominantly white, middle-class area to a skid-row clinic, he found that almost all the improvements available from evening primrose oil and its accessory nutrients could be induced in his new clients (who could not afford such luxuries) *simply by withdrawing certain foods*. It seems that what you don't eat is quite as important as what you do eat.

## PROBLEM FOODS

The foods which caused most symptoms in an American population of food-allergic people were as follows:**

| | | | |
|---|---|---|---|
| Cow's milk | 59% | Potato | 37% |
| Wheat | 55% | Onions | 36% |
| Coffee | 45% | Sugar | 35% |
| Cottage cheese | 38% | Peanuts | 35% |
| Corn | 38% | Beef | 33% |

Their symptoms included depression, indigestion, diarrhoea, irritability, fatigue, clouded thinking, food craving, insomnia, headache, sinus congestion, runny nose and anxiety. Is it a coincidence that TV commercials bombard us with remedies for

*This study is a case-history of an atopic child whose serious allergy to peanuts turned into life-threatening anaphylactic shock after taking aspirin. Thirty minutes after aspirin is taken, absorption of substances with molecular weights up to 70,000 is greatly increased.

**Yeast, fermented foods and drinks, mushrooms and tannin also appear often on such lists.

these very problems, or are functional EFA deficiencies, and therefore food allergies, epidemic amongst us?

## DR ROBERT CATHCART STRIKES AGAIN

Dr Cathcart* points out that stress, toxins, poor diet, allergic reactions and other aspects of modern life all deplete antioxidants such as vitamin C and selenium[86]. According to Cathcart, the resulting more oxidizing conditions sensitize antibodies. This interesting idea could explain why *stress makes allergies worse, and why large doses of vitamin C can alleviate allergic reactions* in some cases**.

Cathcart believes that a normal immune system uses this effect to its advantage. In healthy tissue with plentiful antioxidants***, antibodies are not very sensitive and ordinary invaders are simply eaten by white cells in the process called 'phagocytosis'. However, more dangerous invaders use free radicals**** to disable the white cells. This uses up local antioxidants, which, according to Cathcart, arouses the second line of defence and *causes the antibodies to wake up and mark the invader for destruction*****. When normal conditions return, the antibodies go

*The vitamin C man from page 133.

**Dr Cathcart uses vitamin C to alleviate his hay fever.

***We lost the ability to make vitamin C from blood sugar about 65 million years ago, although other primates did not. Perhaps our diet contained radical quantities of vitamin C at the time. Probably pre-humans could modulate their immune response to avoid auto-immunity, but the stresses of modern living clearly put this goal beyond our reach if we eat a modern, antioxidant-poor diet.

****'Respiratory bursts' of free radicals are a kind of lethal bad breath employed by both invading cells and some immune system white cells to zap each other. More on free radicals on page 74.

*****This is a very easy hypothesis to test. Vitamin C is oxidized to dehydroascorbic acid, and the ratio of C to dehydro-C gives a picture of the oxidizing-reducing balance. Normally about 14, this ratio in patients who would survive was 0.7 in meningitis, 1.1 in pneumonia and 1.3 in typhoid; if it went below 0.5, the patient died (B. Chakrabarti, 'Dehydroascorbic Acid Level in Blood of Patients Suffering from Various Diseases', *P.S.E.B.M.*, 1955, 88:581-583). Tests for C today lump C and dehydro-C together, which can give a profoundly misleading total in infection.

back to sleep, which is just what you need to avoid auto-immune reactions.

However, many aspects of modern life such as air pollution, stress and even painkillers increase our need for antioxidants. Coupled with our poorly chosen diets which cause immune-system over-activity*, the stage is set for both auto-immune and food-allergy reactions.

It may be that, in food-allergy reactions, free radicals generated by immune-system activity deplete bloodstream antioxidants such as the vitamin C needed for PGE1 production. *This could explain Dr Bates's observation that food allergies work against the benefits of the **Food for Vitality** programme.*

## GLA Leads To A Progressive Improvement?

Although large quantities of antioxidants plus GLA to protect the gut seem to start a progressive improvement, removing the offending foods is clearly more desirable. The immune system has a very long memory, so minor reactions to these foods may continue for a long time, causing discomfort and lessening the effectiveness of the immune system.

Unfortunately, the usual battery of tests used by allergists don't identify most damaging foods because these tests are geared to detecting immediate, immunoglobulin-E-allergic reactions.

So how do you know if you're allergic to a food? Generally, such foods are eaten every day, and most will appear in the list on page 154. A sure way to know is to switch

*To be more precise, our poorly chosen diets may not only be low in antioxidants, they also induce functional EFA deficiencies (with their content of, for example, saturated fat and hydrogenates) which results in low PGE1 levels. Since the T-suppressor cells of the immune system seem to be controlled by PGE1, this means that the immune system is more likely to attack indiscriminately, so there will be undesirable food-allergy and auto-immune reactions.

from your usual fare to foods which most people are not allergic*.

## SAFER FOODS

FISH, MOLLUSCS, CRUSTACEANS
LAMB, VEAL, VENISON
VEGETABLES
BROWN RICE
BEANS
FRUIT
EXCEPTION: ANY FOODS HABITUALLY EATEN

After the four days or so that it takes to get foods completely out of the system, add back foods from your usual diet one at a time, watching carefully for reactions. This sounds simple, but the four days are often profoundly unpleasant, and symptoms often worsen before improving. Remember that if you have one food allergy, you probably have several.

Books on allergy and food addiction which explain this procedure in greater detail abound. I particularly like *The Type 1/Type 2 Allergy Relief Program*** and Robert Buist's *Food Intolerance****.

Treating yourself for food allergies is desperately difficult. Few have the self-discipline necessary to put aside their favourite foods for unfamiliar foods, and to keep the necessary food diary for

***Muscle testing* is another way of testing for food allergies (also something of a parlour game!). The idea is that, even though we don't know which foods are bad for us, lower centres do know and affect muscular strength. The tester pushes down on your wrist briefly but firmly while your arm is held out sideways at shoulder height (your shoulder joint should remain locked). Repeat the process with a suspect food in your other hand. If the food has a bad effect, your weakened muscles cannot keep your shoulder locked against the push. This is not a trial of strength, and only your shoulder muscles should be involved. Amazingly, muscle testing has a prolific literature: J. Diamond, *Your Body Doesn't Lie*, Warner, NY, 1983; T. Valentine et al., *Applied Kinesiology*, Thorsons, 1987; W. Fischman et al., *Muscle Response Testing*, Richard Marek, NY, 1979, etc.

**Dr Alan Levin and Merla Zellerbach, *The Type 1/Type 2 Allergy Relief Program*, Berkeley, New York, 1983

***Robert Buist, *Food Intolerance*, Prism Press, Sherborne, Dorset, 1984

long enough to get results. However, there are people experienced in this approach (especially practitioners of 'clinical ecology'), but it's best to ask around until you find someone who gets results. This is an area of bizarre notions and little agreement.

## ANTI-FOOD-ALLERGY MEASURES

Interestingly, bicarbonate often cuts food-allergy reactions short, which probably accounts for the immense popularity of antacids such as Alka-Seltzer*. Other anti-food-allergy measures include digestive enzymes or pancreatin, vitamin C, synthetic PGE1 marketed as the prescription drug Cytotec, and Nalcrom, a prescription drug shown to help adverse reactions to foods[87].

*If you do not gain the benefits of the* **Food for Vitality** *programme in full measure, suspect food allergies.*

# *Heart Disease*

***A man is as old as his arteries.***

ELIE METCHNIKOFF (*1845–1916*)

Heart disease exacts an incredible toll. The *annual* US mortality from heart and blood vessel diseases of just under a million people exceeds the *total* death toll of US soldiers killed in the two World Wars, Korea and Vietnam combined!

## ARE YOU AT RISK?

Quinke's pulse test dates from the days of 'horse and buggy' medicine, but it gives a clear indication of the state of your capillaries. Squeeze a fingertip so that the nail bed is white when you release it. If the nail takes longer than a second or so to

*Food allergy reactions inhibit pancreatic secretions, so that stomach acid remains un-neutralized and the kidneys must dump minerals such as calcium, magnesium and zinc to control acidosis. *Several of these minerals are key co-factors for PGE1 production.* Insulin is another pancreatic secretion which is inhibited by food allergies, and some believe that this can be a cause of diabetes (W. Philpott and D. Kalita, *Victory Over Diabetes*, Keats, New Canaan CT, 1983).

become pink again, a diet and exercise programme may be needed to improve your circulation.

In relation to heart disease, everybody knows:

1. High cholesterol, overweight, smoking and high blood pressure are risk factors for heart disease.
2. Faulty diets containing saturated fat and cholesterol-rich foods raise cholesterol levels.
3. Exercise is good for you.
4. Aspirin lowers heart attack risk.
5. Fibre, polyunsaturates and niacin lower cholesterol.

Unfortunately, some of this conventional wisdom may be only partly true.

When I spoke at a continuing-education class for doctors here in Los Angeles, I learned from the other speakers that although screening tests find many people at high risk*, their cholesterol levels often stay stubbornly high in spite of treatment. Even more frustrating, the tests miss about one in five of people who eventually have heart attacks.

These were doctors in practice, not researchers, and I learned that *practising doctors are not exposed to the latest research findings*. The material in my lecture about damaged essential fatty acids and heart attacks was unknown to most of them, and they were fascinated by it. In turn, I was riveted by what I learned from them about the risk factors for heart disease. Together, it seemed, we could begin to understand why almost *half* of all Westerners die from circulatory diseases**, while virtually

*Nearly three-quarters of people over 65 have atherosclerosis bad enough to see with ultrasound in their carotid (neck) arteries, and 10% have greater than 50% blockage. Once there's plaque in the carotid artery, it's already in the coronary arteries, so these people have heart attacks just waiting to happen. Contrary to popular belief, your risk of heart attack is *twice* as high at 70 than it is at 50 years of age (B. Liebman, 'The HDL/Triglycerides Trap', *Nutrition Action Newsletter*, 17(7):5-7. Much of this information is from Dr William Castelli, Director of the Framingham Study which has followed up 5,200 residents of Framingham, Massachusetts, since 1948).

**Diseases of the circulation include heart attack, stroke, phlebitis (the blockage of an artery by a clot) and pulmonary embolism.

nobody will die from this cause in the undeveloped nations*.

## Essential Fatty Acids In Body Fat

Low levels of linoleic acid in body fat** is a good predictor of both high cholesterol level and the likelihood of a heart attack. This is particularly interesting because low LA in babies' body fat increases their appetites enormously (in a quest to find more LA, perhaps?), and is also a characteristic of fat people. Overweight is, of course, a risk for heart disease.

In America, a public health campaign to replace saturated fat with vegetable oils boosted LA in the American diet, and heart attacks diminished as the percentage of LA in American body fat increased. Here in the UK, as the graphs opposite show, there is no such campaign and heart attacks remain at a high level.

## Why *Do* Polyunsaturates Lower Cholesterol?

One reason was advanced by Dr Hugh Sinclair*** as long ago as 1956[88]. He noticed that rats fed fat-free diets tended to deposit cholesterol in skin, but rats who got plentiful linoleic acid from vegetable oils had no such problem. Carbohydrate is easily converted to *oleic* acid in the body if dietary EFAs are low, and cholesterol *oleate* is much harder to transport than the cholesterol *linoleate* formed when linoleic acid is available.

*The one billion Westerners have all the heart attacks, while the other 4 billion people on the Earth are immune!

**Turnover of body fat LA takes about a year, and the composition of body fat reflects the amount of LA in the diet quite closely.

***Dr Hugh Sinclair died peacefully on 22 June 1990, aged 80. His 1956 letter to the *Lancet* commenced interest in the cardiovascular and health effects of the essential fatty acids. He spent the remainder of his life researching the subject, often at his own expense. He made the experiment of eating an Eskimo diet for three months to investigate the effect on non-Eskimos, and an obituary contained the line: 'This was typical of Sinclair: a bold idea, careful planning, self-experimentation with some danger, dilatory publication and a striking conclusion – in this case that the long-chain fatty acids of fish reduce platelet aggregation and are of the greatest importance in diminishing the prevalence of coronary thrombosis' (B. Lloyd, *Lancet*, 336:303, 1990).

## US Heart Attacks and Body Fat LA ...

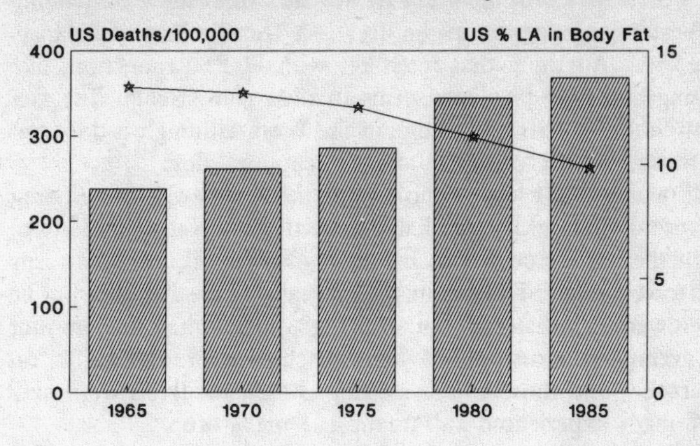


## ... compared with the UK

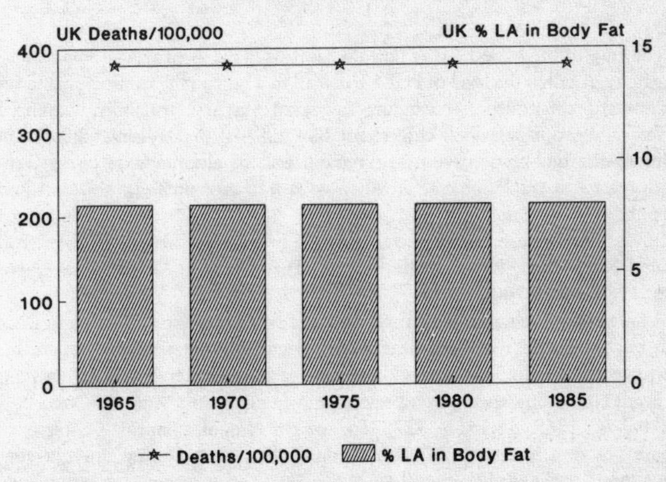


*Figure 8 UK and USA Levels of Body Fat Linoleic Acid Compared*

*The bars show body-fat linoleic acid for Americans and Britons and the lines show the corresponding heart-attack death rates. Notice how the rising LA content of American body fat coincides with their falling death rate, and how both our LA and death rate have remained constant.*

The complementary idea which is slowly emerging is that the EFA derivative *prostaglandin E1* acts as a messenger, controlling cholesterol production in the liver (see The Cholesterol Balance, page 91). Anything that interferes with PGE1 production, like ageing and high-fat diets, seems to raise cholesterol*. The fact that cholesterol rises with age in the West, although it does not in those who eat 'primitive' diets**, supports this.

If raising PGE1 lowers cholesterol, then giving GLA as evening primrose oil should be much more effective at lowering cholesterol than the linoleic acid (LA) in, say, safflower oil, and this turns out to be the case. Three grams of LA added to the diet as vegetable oil lowered cholesterol about 1.5 mg%, while the same amount of evening primrose oil*** lowered cholesterol 30.4 mg%, on average – and those whose starting cholesterol levels were over 308 mg% experienced a dramatic 125 mg% drop[89].

Thus, evening primrose oil GLA was about 163 times more effective than vegetable oil LA in lowering cholesterol****,

*'The core of the hypothesis is that the level of PGE1 is of crucial importance to the body. A fall in the level of PGE1 will lead to a potentially catastrophic series of untoward consequences including increased vascular reactivity, enhanced platelet aggregation, elevated cholesterol biosynthesis, diabetogenic changes in insulin release and responsiveness, enhanced risk of auto-immune disease, enhanced release of arachidonic acid, enhanced risk of inflammatory disorders and susceptibility to depression' (D.F. Horrobin, 'A New Concept of Lifestyle-related Cardiovascular Disease: the Importance of the Interactions between Cholesterol, Essential Fatty Acids, Prostaglandin E1 and Thromboxane A2', *Medical Hypotheses*, 1980, 6:785-800).

**Cholesterol levels hardly change with age in the Japanese, who experience about one fourth the American heart attack death rate. Interestingly, Americans experience a fall in linoleic acid with age, while Japanese levels remain constant (W. Insull et al., 'Studies of Arteriosclerosis in Japanese and American men I', *J. Clin. Invest.*, 1969, 48:1313-1327). To give an idea of a 'normal' cholesterol suppose you're a Kalahari bushman roaming the desert. During drought conditions, your cholesterol level will be about 110, and in times of plenty it may soar to 120 or more (A. Truswell et al., 'Serum-Lipids in Bushmen', *Lancet*, 21 September 1968). In contrast, the average cholesterol level for Westerners is over 200.

***Three grams of evening primrose oil contains 0.36 grams of GLA.

****Efamol* has little effect if cholesterol levels are below about 192 mg/100ml (5 mmol/l). D.F. Horrobin, 'How Do Polyunsaturated Fatty Acids Lower Plasma Cholesterol?', *Lipids,* 18(8):558-562 (1983).

making it *the most potent cholesterol-lowering agent known.* This makes it all the more puzzling that most doctors don't know it exists!

## 'GOOD' HDL (HIGH DENSITY LIPOPROTEIN) CHOLESTEROL*

Evening primrose oil lowers 'bad' LDL (Low Density Lipoprotein which transports cholesterol from the liver to the arteries), and preserves levels of protective, cholesterol-scavenging HDL which takes excess cholesterol back to the liver to be excreted.

This is extremely important because *lowering cholesterol gives no protection if HDL is low*[90]. The *cholesterol-to-HDL* ratio is a much more sensitive predictor of heart attack risk than cholesterol by itself, and low HDL may be one reason why as many as 20% of heart attack victims have cholesterol below the supposedly safe 200 mg% level.

## CHOLESTEROL-TO-HDL RATIO VALUES

| | |
|---|---|
| Safe region**. Atherosclerosis probably *regresses* here | less than 3.5 |
| Atherosclerosis progresses slowly but heart attack risk is low | 3.5 to 4.5 |
| Rapid progression of atherosclerosis with danger of heart attack | over 4.5 |

*Cholesterol is carried from the liver as LDL. Delivering cholesterol to the tissues raises LDL's density so it becomes HDL, which should deliver any excess back to the liver. Unfortunately, if the essential fatty acid metabolism is askew, the liver makes *too much* LDL. Other cholesterol-containing blood components include the *triglycerides* which deliver fats and oils for the tissues to use or burn for calories. Triglycerides above 150 are dangerous if HDL is below 40 – alcohol and refined carbohydrates raise triglycerides, while fish oils lower them.

**A cholesterol level of less than 150 gives apparent immunity from heart attacks, as well as cancer of the breast and colon, and Type II diabetes. An HDL over 60 also seems to give complete protection from heart attacks, while an HDL of less than 35 means grave danger, whatever the cholesterol level.

## CHOLESTEROL-LOWERING DRUGS

*If the whole materia medica as now used could be sunk to the bottom of the sea, it would be all the better for mankind – and all the worse for the fishes.*

OLIVER WENDELL HOLMES, MD

Interestingly, the oestrogen used in hormone-replacement therapy raises HDL and cuts heart attack risk by two-thirds in post-menopausal women*, although smoking cancels this effect. The drug gemfibrozil (Lopid) lowered heart attack risk by 34% in one study and two-thirds of this lowered risk was due to raised HDL[91], but Lopid's side-effects are similar to other cholesterol-lowerers and include tummy troubles, fatigue, headaches and liver damage[92]. Other cholesterol-lowering drugs have horrific side-effects, including loss of sexual desire and increased risk of suicide. The popular self-help 'natural' cholesterol remedy, niacin or vitamin $B_6$, unfortunately *raises* insulin resistance when given in quantities large enough to lower cholesterol, causing the characteristic spare tyre or apple-pattern of overweight[93]. So perhaps the best cholesterol-lowering 'drug' of all is exercise, which both lowers 'bad' LDL and raises 'good' HDL.

## THE IMPORTANCE OF EXERCISE

Nathan Pritikin astonished the medical profession by showing that exercise and a very low-fat diet saves lives and rehabilitates heart-attack victims. The condition of his own heart at his death in 1985 prompted his pathologists to write that 'in a man 69 years old [who was diagnosed with severe atherosclerosis in 1958], the near absence of atherosclerosis and the complete absence of its effects are remarkable'[94]**.

*Atherosclerosis proceeds at the same pace in post-menopausal women as it does in men but heart attack risk rises faster, perhaps because women's arteries are so much smaller than men's.

**The Pritikin diet and exercise programme is a life-saver for the gravely ill – a perfect antidote for a life-time high-fat Western diet – but it places terrible demands on reserves of the essential fatty acids. Pritikin himself died of malignant lymphoma, a condition he already had when he was diagnosed with severe atherosclerosis in 1958. Was his diet unable to protect him against cancer because it's so low in essential fatty acids?

The biggest benefit from exercise apparently comes from the first 1500 calories burned per week. This means half-an-hour's brisk walking or aerobics, a 5-mile bicycle ride or swimming 800 yards *each day*. Such a programme apparently boosts the efficiency of the 'delicate first step' enzyme and restores the essential fatty acid metabolism, for most of its positive effects (such as improved mood, weight loss and lowered cholesterol) complement those of dietary measures which revive the essential fatty acid-to-prostaglandin pathway. For this reason, *you will not get the full benefit of your dietary improvements unless you exercise.*

## Back To Cholesterol-Lowering Dietary Improvements

Cholesterol itself inhibits the 'delicate first step' enzyme, so high cholesterol may cause even higher cholesterol! A way out of this vicious circle is to lower fat and cholesterol in the diet and supply the EFA derivatives ready-made, as in, for example, fish and evening primrose oil. Other foods which change cholesterol levels fall in with this concept:

| *Foods That Raise Cholesterol* | *Foods That Lower Cholesterol* |
|---|---|
| Apple pie | Apples |
| Bacon | Sweetbreads (brains) |
| Beef | Salmon |
| Cheese | Lobster |
| Chocolate Digestives | Crispbreads (Ryvita) |
| Saturated fat | Flaxseed oil (unprocessed) |
| Hydrogenated margarines | Safflower oil (cold-pressed) |
| Supermarket eggs | Liver |
| White bread | Whole-grain bread |

The list suggests that plenty of polyunsaturates in wholefoods with little other fat will lower cholesterol. There is, however, one catch: *not all polyunsaturates are cholesterol-lowering essential oils.*

Most supermarket oils and margarines have low EFA activity because of refining and hydrogenation. The damaged essential fatty acids – 'trans' fats – actually interfere with EFA processing, exerting an 'anti-essential-fatty acid' effect in the body.

## DOES HYDROGENATION ACTUALLY *CAUSE* HEART ATTACKS?

The graph of heart deaths and heart attacks in America, plotted with the percentage of trans fats in American food (see below) has profound implications[95].

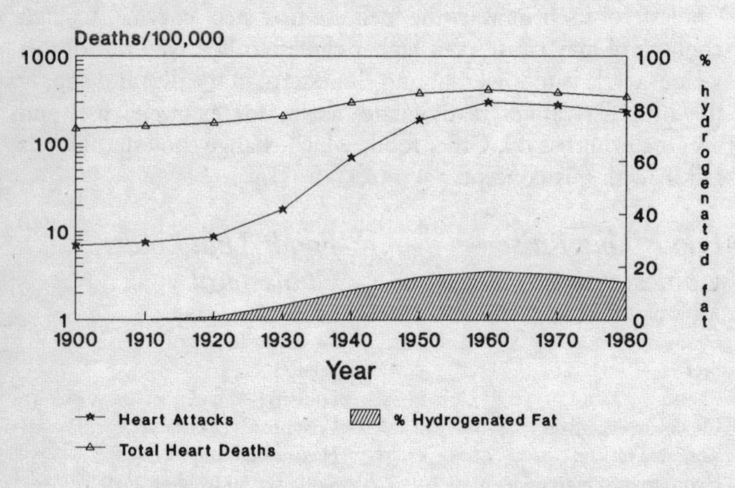


*Figure 9 Hydrogenation and Heart Attacks*

*Hydrogenated fats entered the US diet in 1911[96] (shading). Notice how heart attacks rose from being about 10% of all heart deaths in 1900 to nearly 90% in 1980[97]. Hydrogenation was the* only *qualitative change in the American diet over these years.*

Margarine was a mixture of animal and vegetable fats and milk solids until, in 1911, Crisco became the first hydrogenated product on the American market. Unappetizing white hydrogenated margarines followed, as the powerful dairy industry lobbied successfully against yellow dyes. But hydrogenated margarines sold better during the Depression because their lower prices weighed heavily against both butter and the original-formula margarines.

Then an extraordinary thing happened. Heart attacks, previously almost unknown (the first heart attack in Scotland occurred in 1928[98]) began killing men in their forties and fifties.

From the turn of the century, congestive heart failure and the other heart ailments had killed old people fairly steadily, while angina* (the closest thing to heart attacks at the time) was responsible for only a small percentage of heart deaths. In other words, there was much atherosclerosis, but few heart attacks. Atherosclerosis happens slowly, allowing alternative pathways – 'collateral circulation' – to develop around blocked coronary arteries, so one can live to a ripe old age (even with angina) unless a blood clot suddenly blocks a narrowed artery and causes a heart attack. But what causes the clot?

## HEART ATTACKS! BUT *HOW*?

A very recent study showed that trans fats in a hydrogenated sunflower seed-olive oil blend (similar to commercial margarine) raised the ratio of cholesterol-to-HDL by 23%, while saturated fat raised it only 13%[99]**. Thus, *margarines are much more*

*After Angina Pectoris, heart attacks were called diseases of the Coronary Arteries, then Arteriosclerotic Heart Disease, and, finally, Ischemic Heart Disease. A review in *The Journal of the American Medical Association* for 1921 barely mentions heart attacks: 'Myocardial infarction from coronary thrombosis, if extensive, [leads] to cardiac aneurysm and perforation into the pericardium, a structural change in the heart which is usually diagnosticated at the necropsy table. There is clinical evidence of the condition, however, on occasion, in the presence of severe prolonged heart pain if the thrombosis is extensive. Arteriosclerosis is the usual etiologic factor.' In other words, people survived heart attacks! At that time, 'Arteriosclerotic Heart Disease or Cardiosclerosis [was] by far the commonest etiologic type of all [heart diseases].' (O. Pepper 'Diseases of the Thorax and its Viscera, Including the Heart, Lungs and Blood Vessels', *JAMA*, 1921, 77:1414)

**HDL is 'good' High Density Lipoprotein which transports cholesterol to the liver, and the ratio is an indicator of heart attack risk.

*dangerous than butter as far as heart attacks are concerned**.

It seems that hydrogenation first destroys the omega-3 ancestor of blood-thinning, clot-busting, artery-dilating 'good guy' prostaglandins (prostacyclin). Then it changes much of the omega-6 LA into the trans form, which baffles the enzymes which try to make it into another 'good guy', prostaglandin E1. Without these 'good guys', the arachidonic acid (AA) from eggs, milk and meat can be made into the artery-constricting, blood-clotting agents of heart attacks – thromboxanes and leukotrienes. In fact, the prostacyclin-thromboxane ratio turns out to be very low in heart attack victims.

Here is a smoking gun, but can we find the bullet? It was found in 1981 and confirmed in 1983 that *heart attack victims had more hydrogenated fats and less animal fat in their bodies than people who died from other causes*[100,101] – so the unfortunate heart attack victims had cut down on animal fats by substituting 'killer' margarine!

Incredibly, *food analysts still lump the trans's together with natural 'cis' essential fatty acids in their dietary analyses*! Ominously, up to 18% trans fats have been found in the milk of nursing mothers[102]**, and our tissues contain up to 12.5% – more if we load up on hydrogenated margarines***.

*As long ago as 1964, an analysis of dietary changes pointed out that heart attacks in white males increased 40% between 1940 and 1954, and that post-mortem clots had increased considerably since 1945, concluding that excessive 'consumption of saturated fat . . . *especially since the introduction of hydrogenated vegetable oils*, is responsible, at least in part, for the increase in coronary heart disease.' M. Antar et al., 'Changes in Retail Market Food Supplies in the United States in the Last Seventy Years in Relation to the Incidence of Coronary Heart Disease', *Am J. Clin. Nutr.* 14:169-178 (1964)

**This is particularly ominous because developing rat brains cannot discriminate between trans and cis fatty acids, and the same is probably true of people (H. Cook, 'Incorporation, Metabolism and Positional Distribution of trans-Unsaturated Fatty Acids in Developing and Mature Brain', *Biochimica et Biophysica Acta.*, 1978, 531:245-256). This 18% trans content of breast milk could explain why 96% of Canadian infants who died accidentally in the first months of life had extensive signs of developing atherosclerosis (D. Jaffe et al., 'Coronary Arteries in Newborn Children', *Act Paed. Scan.*, 1971, Suppl. 219)

***Estimates vary from 12 grams/day (M. Enig, *Federation Proceedings*, 1978, 37:2215-2220) to 20 grams/day (J. Booyens et al., *Medical Hypotheses*, 1986, 21:387-408).

Traditional-living Eskimos, who are virtually immune from heart attacks, have none – their diet is mostly fish and seal meat and contains no processed fats.

So what emerges from all this is that low LA in body fat lowers prostaglandin protection into heart-attack territory, more so when trans fats are present. That Glaswegians with the same degree of atherosclerosis as Londoners had many more heart attacks supports this view[103], for margarine consumption is rather higher, and vegetable oil (LA) consumption rather lower, in Scotland.

It seems that cholesterol-lowering gives no safety unless HDL is high – in other words, *protection from heart attacks comes from a working essential fatty acid metabolism.* Using drugs or any other method may mitigate heart disease *but leaves the person open to all the other diseases of disturbed essential fatty acid derivatives listed on page 113.*[104]

## THE IMPORTANCE OF FISH*

One consistent observation in heart attack research is that a little fish goes a long way towards protection from heart attack risk. Thus, in 1985, Dr Kromhout found just 35 grams of fish per day (about one third of an average serving) halved heart attack deaths[105], and this has been amply confirmed by a wealth of studies since[106]**.

Fish oils show up in platelets, the part of the blood most involved in clotting. A high content of the fish oil EPA makes platelets much less inclined to clot by discouraging thromboxane and encouraging prostacyclin formation. Fish almost always lowers triglycerides, and usually lowers cholesterol.

*Cold-water ocean fish, that is. The distressing tendency for fish farms to feed sewage-sludge pellets and other foods low in omega-3 essential fatty acids means that much fish-farmed fish may be without value against heart ailments. However, Norwegian salmon is often fish-farmed in fjords, and is probably OK.

**A 100g serving of mackerel or salmon contains about 2 grams of omega-3s, and this amount proved best for reducing 'bad' LDL and triglyceride levels and raising HDL. In the American population, *the study found no benefit from increased consumption beyond this level* (*American Journal of Clinical Nutrition*, 1990, 52(1):120).

## Avoid Fish Oil Supplements

However, taking fish oil *supplements* may not accomplish the same goal. Studies have found, for example, that high doses* of fish oil supplements can raise LDL (bad) cholesterol[107], that they are helpless to prevent opened-up coronary arteries from blocking up again[108] and that they cause insulin resistance in diabetics[109].

These bad effects may be because *too much* fish oil inhibits processing of the omega-6 family of EFAs, lowering GLA and lessening PGE1 production – and low PGE1 for whatever reason is very bad news. How much is too much? We don't know, but we do know that eating cold-water fish is protective, and that *protection starts with just two fish meals per week*.

A second reason *not* to megadose with fish oil supplements is that such oils require antioxidant protection, and too much fish oil may outstrip the capacity of bloodstream vitamin C. Oxidation promotes free radical activity and causes all sorts of problems, such as damaging the arterial lining[110] and lessening protective prostacyclin production[111]**.

A respected heart-disease researcher summed up prevailing opinion when he wrote that 'If you eat a small quantity of oily fish every day, say a minimum of 30g/1 oz of mackerel or the equivalent in any other fish, you do not need supplements.'[112]

If you can't stand fish in any form, then avoid supplements processed to provide higher levels of EPA and DHA. They haven't performed well in studies, and we evidently don't know enough yet to be able to outperform Mother Nature. Take unmodified fish oil such as cod liver oil.

## The Importance of Antioxidants

Vitamin C has a property which is extremely valuable to those at risk from heart attack. Diseased arteries produce less and less

*At 12–15 capsules a day, equivalent to a Greenland Eskimo's intake, 'good' HDL remained constant but 'bad' LDL increased 16%.

**Although one research team suggests that fish oil's good effect actually *stems* from free radical activity inhibiting 'Platelet Derived Growth Factor c' which makes atherosclerotic plaque worse! (J. Raloff, 'A Radical Role For Dietary Fish Oils', *Science News*, 1988, 134(4):52)

prostacyclin, the prostaglandin which keeps them slippery and free of clots, but *taking vitamin C encourages prostacyclin production even when atherosclerosis is far advanced*[113].

The reason probably has to do with vitamin C's antioxidant property of neutralizing free radicals*, which has another benefit. Vitamin C is the *only* antioxidant capable of fully protecting the cholesterol and fatty acids in Low Density Lipoproteins[114]**, albeit at higher levels than those necessary to prevent scurvy which is a strong argument in favour of raising the Recommended Dietary Allowance. Oxidized cholesterol and lipid peroxides damage the arterial lining, and some believe that this is the first step in the development of atherosclerosis[115].

A vitamin C researcher, Dr Emil Ginter, points out that the decline in heart deaths in the United States bears an inverse relation to vitamin C production***. It seems that, over time, vitamin C lowers cholesterol levels in those under 25, and protects against strokes and heart attacks (and recurrences) in old people****. The mechanism is probably partly enhanced by PGE1 production, since vitamin C is necessary for steps between DGLA and PGE1. Dr Constance Spittle of Pinderfields Hospital in Yorkshire, who noticed vitamin C's cholesterol-lowering effect, suggests half a gram per day for normal young people, and up to 3 grams for older people[116].

Beta-carotene, another antioxidant, has been shown to slow the progression of heart disease by the same team who found aspirin to be protective against heart attacks (page 49)[117].

*Lipid peroxides – rancid fats – in the bloodstream generate free radical activity which reduce prostacyclin production ('Prostacyclin and Atherosclerosis', *Human Pathology* 1985, 16(3):201)

**The villainous LDLs associated with increased heart attack risk.

***Ginter believes that C activates the liver enzyme responsible for bile production (E. Ginter, 'Decline of Coronary Mortality in United States and Vitamin C', *Am. J. Clin. Nutr.*, 1979, 32(3):511-512).

****The burns unit of Pinderfields Hospital routinely gave 1 gram of C daily to help recovery. After 6 years, somebody noticed there had been but one fatal pulmonary embolism and no deep-vein thrombosis. This is an incredible record. ('A Vitamin Answer to Atherosclerosis?' *Medical World News*, 13 September 1974, p. 64G).

# Avoid Aspirin

When the Reverend Edward Stone demonstrated to the Royal Society in 1763 that an extract of willow bark* controlled fever, he showed that aspirin, like too much fish oil, shuts down the prostaglandin metabolism. However, *this only helps matters when the prostaglandin metabolism is deranged***. Boosting prostacyclin and lowering thromboxane with fish, evening primrose oil and so forth is infinitely preferable to taking aspirin. Aspirin throws the baby out with the bath water because *certain prostaglandins promote healing****.

This is nowhere more apparent than in rheumatoid arthritis. *Long-term use of prostaglandin-inhibiting anti-inflammatories is associated with joint deterioration*, just as one might expect[118]. What, then, is aspirin's long-term effect on the coronary arteries? It is unlikely to be good, and since everything that aspirin can do

*Willow bark contains salicylates which are natural forms of aspirin.

**Aspirin became big news when the 1988 Physicians' Health Study revealed that 325 mg every other day cut heart attack risk by 47% in 22,000 male physicians. In the British Radcliffe Infirmary study which followed almost immediately, five thousand doctors took 500 mg and found only a 30% reduction in risk (*Science News*, 1988, 133(5):68 and 133(6):84). The solution to the puzzle may be that 325 mg every other day knocks out *prostaglandin* production in the platelets, which lessens clotting, while 500 mg may be enough to knock out some of the enzymes which make beneficial *prostacyclin* in the blood vessel wall as well. It's encouraging that this *selective* inhibition of prostaglandins is the first advance on Reverend Stone's 1763 shotgun approach, but consider that mortality among the physicians was 189 fatal heart attacks in the control group and 104 in the aspirin group. When you consider that there wouldn't have been *any* heart attacks in Stone's time, it's clear that there *has* to be a better mousetrap.

***Leaf and Webber wrote that 'aspirin . . . is prescribed only to block the platelet production of thromboxane, whereas n-3 fatty acids interfere with the pathological developments in atherosclerosis at several loci. Thus, n-3 fatty acids may have more clinical benefits than aspirin, even though aspirin is a more effective inhibitor of thromboxane synthesis.' (Cardiovascular Effects of the n-3 Fatty Acids, *New Eng. J. Med.*, 1988, 318(9):549-557). Aspirin can cause gastric bleeding, depress immune function and heighten stroke risk. In contrast, essential fatty acid therapy not only controls clotting better than aspirin, it also causes vasodilation, increases red cell deformability, reduces cholesterol and lessens hypertension.

can be accomplished with diet and exercise, the aspirin experiment is best left to others*.

The best strategy for avoiding heart problems is, then, to take steps to maximize PGE1 production – in other words, to follow the dietary principles set out in this book.

Now we can add some **extra points** to the conventional wisdom already mentioned at the beginning of this section:

1. High cholesterol, overweight, smoking and high blood pressure are risk factors for heart disease.
2. Faulty diets containing saturated fat and cholesterol-rich foods raise cholesterol levels.
3. Exercise is good for you.
4. Healthy levels of High Density Lipoproteins are a must, and seem to stem from a working essential fatty acid-to-prostaglandin pathway.
5. Aspirin interferes with healing because it cancels the good prostaglandins as well as the inflammatory varieties, *so it only helps when the EFAs are disordered*. It makes much more sense to correct the esssential fatty acids in the diet and avoid aspirin completely.
6. Avoiding foods high in AA such as milk, meat and eggs may lower 'bad' inflammatory AA derivatives**.
7. Fibre, essential fatty acids (as in cold-pressed, unrefined flax-seed and safflower seed oils) and vitamins C, $B_6$, $B_3$ and the minerals zinc, copper, chromium and magnesium all help lower cholesterol.
8. These steps, along with evening primrose oil and cold-water fish, should correct the disturbed pattern of essential fatty acid

*Apparently, aspirin affords little or no protection over what you get from fish oil (E. van den Berg et al., 'Hemostatic Function in Patients Receiving n-3 Fatty Acids in Addition to Anti-Platelet Agents', *Clin. Res.*, 35:7A).

**Thromboxanes, leukotrienes and 2-series prostaglandins.

derivatives found in atherosclerosis, thin the blood and lower cholesterol and triglyceride levels.

Do all this, and you may outlive your doctor!

## *High Blood Pressure*

Hypertension predisposes to heart disease and is an all-around Bad Thing. One in ten of us has it, and the incidence rises sharply after 45 years of age. Among more traditional-living peoples, there is no such age-related rise in blood pressure, and neither do their body-fat linoleic acid (LA) levels fall with age as ours do*.

Dr Peter Oster studied 650 German men and found that the lower their body-fat LA, the higher their blood pressure, cholesterol and body weight[119]. Another study, of 399 Americans with plentiful LA, found a strong connection with body-fat linolenic acid[120]**. (LNA). Numerous other studies suggest that these are not just things that change at the same time, but rather that the rising blood pressure is in some way *caused* by the falling body-fat LA.

Most arachidonic acid derivatives such as prostaglandin E2 and thromboxane A2 raise blood pressure by constricting blood vessels, while prostaglandin E1 and prostacyclin lower it. Thus, both omega-3 oils[121] and the GLA in evening primrose oil[122] should tend to lower blood pressure because they promote PGE1 production and reduce AA derivatives. This prediction was shown to be correct in a study of hypertensives given either flaxseed oil or *Efamol Marine*, which contains both GLA and EPA – those given *Efamol Marine* had significant lowering of their blood pressure. The fact that those given flaxseed oil did not suggest that impaired 'delicate first step' enzyme activity in the EFA-to-prostaglandin pathway caused the high blood pressure in the first place[123].

*Americans' body-fat LA fell from 12% at 20 years of age to 9% at 55 years (W. Insull, 'Studies of Arteriosclerosis in Japanese and American Men 1', *J. Clin. Investigation*, 1969, 48:1313- 1327).

**At 16% LA and 2% LNA, the Americans had 33% more LA and considerably lower blood pressure than the Germans, but Dr Oster did not measure German LNA levels.

## The Effect Of Stress

Stress can turn borderline high blood pressure into hypertension, but a study has shown that the GLA in borage seed oil* blocks this effect, both in rats bred to develop hypertension and in people[124]. Interestingly, the researchers wrote that 60% of the people in the borage oil group in this double-blind study spontaneously reported either feeling better, lessened anxiety or that they could concentrate better, but there were no such comments from those taking placebos in the control group.

## Vitamin C, Again

High blood levels of vitamin C were associated with normal blood pressure in both healthy Americans and elderly Chinese-Americans, while low levels were associated with higher blood pressure[125]. The researchers thought that perhaps the vitamin C was preventing artery damage from free radicals but it seems more likely that it was promoting artery-relaxing PGE1 production.

## Raw Foods And Blood Pressure

Dr John Douglass of Los Angeles noticed that people who ate plenty of raw vegetables had low blood pressure[126]. He tested the idea on 32 of his patients (28 of whom were obese) by suggesting that at least 40% of their diets should consist of uncooked foods such as vegetables, seeds, nuts, fruits, seed oil and raw milk. After six months, they were eating about 62% of their food raw, and had lost up to 6.4 kg and an average of 18 points from their blood pressure[127]**. Some of the reasons for this effect are discussed on page 63.

It seems that both overweight and high blood pressure can be the end-result of many different problems. Misery, eating disorders, metabolic disturbances, inactive brown fat and mineral-poor diets are just a few of the possible reasons. However, raising

*Evening primrose oil is probably more effective – see page 101.

**The mean diastolic pressure reduction was 18 mm Hg which was statistically significant (P<.00001).

the amount of EFAs in the body-fat by eating close to the ***Food for Vitality*** programme seems to affect the mechanisms which actually *cause* the body to put on fat. In fact, Dr Douglass believes that six months on a fairly raw diet will solve almost any high blood pressure problem.

## *Hyperactivity*

Children with severe 'Attention Deficit Disorder' seem wildly over-stimulated and can't sit still or concentrate on anything for more than a few seconds. Attempts at discipline lead to hysterical outbursts or tantrums, and sleep is interrupted by frequent nightmares (even when exhausted). Demands must be met immediately, but the child seems able to take little pleasure in anything. There is compulsive aggression and disruption both at school and at home, which cannot be prevented with even the harshest punishment.

Nobody can deal with this problem alone. Hyperactive children are flat-out unlovable. If you have such a child, join the Hyperactive Children's Support Group*. Their diet and supplement programme is thoroughly practical, developed of necessity by parents of hyperactive children. If anybody knows what works, they do.

An HACSG survey of 102 hyperactive children indicates that most (92%) have an atopic background, and that one third of them (34%) have either eczema or asthma, or both. Most are boys. All this puts the condition squarely in the 'disturbed EFA derivative' category, and low levels of DGLA have been confirmed in hyperactive children[128]. However, initial studies seemed to show that GLA supplementation is not a panacea[129].

Typically, of 85 hyperactive children, the 31% 'classical' hyperactives (without atopy) didn't respond at all, and, of the remainder, 18% improved slightly and 44% improved a lot[130]**. Those who improved somewhat had atopic backgrounds, but those who got much better *had family members with histories of*

*The Hyperactive Children's Support Group, 71 Whyke Lane, Chichester, West Sussex PO19 2LD.

**Only 1% got worse, but 7% failed to complete the study. Their parents were unwilling to switch to the placebo!

*mood swings, and drug or alcohol abuse.* The emphasis draws attention to the fact that these conditions, like atopy, involve essential fatty acid disturbances.

Hyperactive children seem to have a lessened ability to convert linoleic acid to GLA, which would account for their low blood levels of derivatives. The Feingold diet* eliminates many mild blockers of essential fatty acid metabolism, such as the natural salicylates found in tomatoes, almonds, apples and cucumbers (among other foods), preservatives and the yellow food dye tartrazine.

The best book that I've seen is *The Hyperactive Child*** by Belinda Barnes and Irene Colquhoun. Belinda Barnes ran Foresight, the Association for Pre-Conceptual Care, and Irene Colquhoun is Chairman of the Hyperactive Children's Parent Support Group.

## THE FEINGOLD DIET

According to the HACSG, the Feingold diet helps 94% of hyperactive children and is the first step in treatment. Their survey also revealed that 78% of hyperactive children have abnormal thirst without increased urine production and that this trait strongly suggests the child will respond to evening primrose oil. Interestingly, this is a marker for essential fatty acid *deficiency*, so it seems likely that the children's EFA-to-prostaglandin pathway defects are made worse by poor absorption, inadequate diet or increased usage of dietary linoleic acid in vegetable oils.

What about the 20–30% who do not respond fully? Firstly, it is highly likely they have deficiencies of nutrients such as zinc, magnesium and vitamins C, $B_3$ or $B_6$ which promote the essential

*The late Dr Ben Feingold developed his diet to treat people with bad allergies, but one patient's severe psychological disturbance also responded. This prompted him to try it on hyperactive children, about 50% of whom recovered and another 20% responded enough to be taken off drugs. The side effects of Ritalin, the usual drug for hyperactivity, include toxic psychosis, anorexia, hypersensitivity reactions (such as hives), hair loss and anaemia, so this is a most valuable contribution. The diet is fully described in his book, *Why your Child is Hyperactive*, Random House, New York, 1974.

**Thorsons, Wellingborough, Northamptonshire, 1984.

fatty acid metabolism. A supplement such as *Optivite* will help here. A related problem is excesses of toxic minerals such as lead and aluminium, which can have profound behavioural effects. These can be tested for by a doctor or holistic practitioner.

Secondly, food allergy to milk products and other foods may well be a factor (see page 151). Eliminating high-risk foods (especially fizzy drinks and junk foods) for a few days will usually identify the foods involved.

Finally, 'chemical hypersensitivity' may contribute. If behaviour deteriorates with exposure to felt-tip pens or other chemicals, then the child may be deficient in selenium. A series of articles in *The International Journal of Bio-Social Research* by Dr Stephen Levine are very informative about this[131]. Dr Levine himself suffered from chemical hypersensitivity, or environmental illness as it is sometimes called, and developed a cure. Reprints of the articles and the sodium selenite solution used to treat it are available from Nutricology*.

# *Irritability, Depression and Manic Depression*

***Every one is more or less mad on one point.***

RUDYARD KIPLING

An unusual effect surfaced in numerous studies of GLA-containing oils such as evening primrose oil. In scientific studies, more people usually drop out of the groups receiving medicine than out of the control groups taking placebos. However, in several GLA trials, drop outs were much higher in the control groups. Active-group subjects often asked what they were taking and where they could get it, saying that it increased their sense of well-being[132]**. *I suspect this feeling of well-being is our natural state*, and our more usual irritable, thin-skinned frame of mind is a consequence of functional EFA deficiency.

*Nutricology Inc., 400 Preda Street, San Leandro, CA 94577-0489, USA. Tel. (415) 639-4572

**For example, see page 175.

## IRRITABILITY AND DEPRESSION

Oddly enough, both irritability and hair-trigger temper are characteristics of depression, and I suspect they are symptoms of low PGE1 and that this book's proposed pattern of eating will help. Whether deranged EFAs heighten sensitivity to hormones, as is thought to happen in PMT, or depression and irritability are simply low-PGE1 symptoms, the effect is clearly present and very widespread.

From my experience, I suspect that alcohol is often a reason that PGE1 is low, so that alcohol is an indirect cause of irritability. When the police respond to 'domestic trouble' calls, alcohol is usually involved. Alcoholics are frequently depressed (see page 118) and alcohol is involved in an impressive proportion of violent incidents. I have seen relationships in which husband and wife apparently hated each other literally transformed when alcohol was withdrawn.

The book to read here is *Essential Fatty Acids in Immunity and Mental Health** by Dr Charles Bates. Dr Bates brings out the inter-relationships between race, essential fatty acid requirement and food allergies. He provides insight into and solutions for practical problems such as marital strife, irritability, depression and chronic fatigue.

## MANIC DEPRESSION

Manic Depression is a devastating condition in which one cycles endlessly between euphoria, which can be so intense as to be psychotic, and immobilizing depression. We don't really know what causes manic depression, but there's a genetic component to it and the psychotic episodes can sometimes be linked to an unpleasant triggering event.

Interestingly, blood platelets from manic depressives produce much more PGE1 when stimulated in the laboratory during the manic phase than they do during depression – see the graph

*Available from Life Science Press, Tacoma, Washington, USA. Tel. (206) 922-0442

opposite. It may seem like two wild leaps of faith to assume firstly that brain PGE1 levels correspond, and secondly that PGE1 affects brain functioning. However, the usual treatment of lithium carbonate, which effectively controls the manic phase and prevents reoccurrences, *stabilizes PGE1 levels*. Interestingly, lithium is plentiful in food at the ocean margin, where Dr Crawford proposes that we evolved.

PGE1 appears to control the T-suppressor cells[133]* of the immune system, so that high PGE1 means high T-suppressor cell activity and a calm immune system, while low PGE1 means inactive T-suppressors and perhaps too much immune activity, as in the auto-immune assault on myelin during MS attacks. *PGE1 is high in euphoria and MS remissions, and low in depression and MS flare-ups*.

Accordingly, Drs David Horrobin and Julian Lieb have suggested that the chronic, remitting inflammatory diseases such as multiple sclerosis, rheumatoid arthritis and atopic asthma may be a kind of *manic depression of the immune system*[134]**.

Lithium may work by regulating PGE1 production, preventing PGE1 over-production in the euphoric phase of manic-depression which quickly exhausts DGLA supplies and triggers a PGE1-deficiency depression. If this is the case, it explains why lithium controls euphoria but has less effect on depression, and also why lithium prevents recurrences of manic euphoria***.

If Drs Horrobin and Lieb are right, not only should lithium either improve or worsen the disturbed-EFA diseases, but the more natural remedy for PGE1 fluctuations of giving GLA in evening primrose oil should help manic-depressives. Much peripheral evidence indicates both predictions are true. Heart disease is inversely proportional to lithium concentration in drinking water[135]. Lithium helped prevent recurrent asthma attacks[136], but

*T-helper cells turn on B-cell antibody production during infections. When the immune system has destroyed the invader, T-suppressors are supposed to close down B-cell antibody production. If they don't, there may be auto-immunity, as in rheumatoid arthritis flare-ups, and if the T-suppressors are too active, the immune system may not react to invaders at all.

**Also Crohn's Disease, Ulcerative Colitis, Migraine and the Collagen Diseases.

***That is, by preventing DGLA exhaustion from PGE1 over-production.

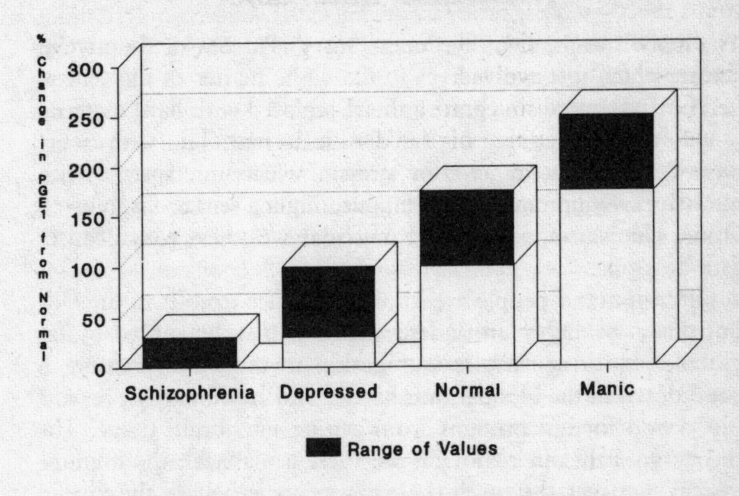


*Figure 10 Prostaglandin E1 and Mood in Illness*

***When blood platelets were stimulated to make PGE1 in the laboratory, depressed and manic patients made quantities which neatly bracketed normal levels. Schizophrenics' platelets made almost none, and no amount of stimulation made schizophrenics' platelets produce anything like normal levels. Figure redrawn from data in reference 133.***

either improved or worsened acne and eczema[137]*. And Dr Lieb has found that *manic depressives who got tremors and dysphoria (felt bad) while on lithium could take it if given plentiful linoleic-acid-containing vegetable oil at the same time*[138].

All this could mean that lithium is an esssential nutrient. Certainly, we were exposed to plenty of it in our evolutionary diet if Dr Crawford is right about where we evolved. Perhaps

*Too much lithium could lower PGE1 too much, causing auto-immunity, while too little might allow PGE1 to reach levels which would prevent the immune system from responding at all.

shellfish, which are rich in lithium, will one day emerge as a treatment for manic depression!

## *Multiple Sclerosis*

The name means, literally, 'many scars'. Patches of the myelin sheath which insulates nerves in the white matter of the central nervous system* disintegrate and are replaced with hard material – scar tissue. Progress of the disease is irregular, with acute phases sometimes triggered by stressful events interspersed with remissions. Symptoms include fatigue, tingling sensations, blurred vision, clumsiness, vertigo and muscular weakness which causes foot-dragging.

Fifty thousand people are known to suffer from it in the UK, but this is probably an underestimate. It may be caused by fat globules blocking venules (capillaries) in the brain, causing a breakdown in the blood–brain barrier which ordinarily prevents blood and foreign proteins from getting into brain tissue. The theory goes that in removing the foreign material, the immune system damages the myelin. However, some believe the myelin itself may be poorly constructed, a consequence of bottle-feeding linoleic-acid-poor cow's milk during development of the nervous system.

Epidemiology tells us that the distribution of MS follows that of heart disease – high in sugar and dairy-consuming areas, low where people eat more fish and vegetable oils. Those most at risk have a congenital oddity in fat-handling called Thompson's anomaly which leaves their red and white blood cells, myelin and blood plasma low in essential fatty acids, especially linoleic acid.

This predisposition can be detected with the 'electrophoretic mobility test', in which red cells' speed of movement is compared in solutions rich in either AA (arachidonic acid) or LA (linoleic acid). Nutritional therapy similar to the diet in this book can return fatty acid profiles and cell mobility towards normal, stabilizing the disease.

*Only the brain and spinal cord are affected. The myelin of the peripheral nervous system contains different proteins.

The best book I've seen on this subject is Judy Graham's *Multiple Sclerosis, A Self-Help Guide to Its Management** – particularly since her dietary suggestions are in line with the ***Food for Vitality*** programme! Judy Graham got MS in 1974 when she was twenty-seven and has held her ground to the present with minimal deterioration. She gave birth to a healthy boy when she was thirty-eight.

## *Osteoporosis*

Rats develop osteoporosis when deprived of essential fatty acids[139], and Dr David Horrobin has suggested that osteoporosis shares characteristics of the functional EFA deficiency diseases[140]. Bone is, of course, connective tissue, and the health of our connective tissues depends on how well our EFA-to-prostaglandin pathways are working. The 'delicate first step' enzyme declines with age first in the testes and lastly in the liver, and this decline may be responsible for many of the changes of ageing. It will be most interesting to see if osteoporosis is one of them.

## *Overweight*

A Ministry of Agriculture, Fisheries and Food survey found nearly *half* the male population of Britain is overweight, and *two-thirds* have a high risk of heart disease![141]

Is obesity a disturbed-EFA disease? Perhaps.

Consider that in a study of blood pressure and body-fat linoleic acid in 650 German men, an incidental finding was that those of normal weight had high LA levels, and vice-versa[142]. Remember that babies' food intakes increased enormously when the EFA content of their formula was reduced, implying that an LA deficiency has an appetite-enhancing effect[143]. Ponder the finding that evening primrose oil activates brown fat[144], the mitochondria-rich fat in the neck and back which burns calories for heat to keep us warm, and burns excess calories to prevent our becoming obese[145].

*Healing Arts Press, Rochester, Vermont, USA, 1989

When normal and obese people were given evening primrose oil in a study, almost all the active group lost weight, although one subject *gained* 6 kg![146]. The results support the idea that evening primrose oil helps *most* people lose weight if they're more than 10% over their ideal weight. Other studies agree[147].

However, the thing that will *really* help weight loss is restoring the essential fatty acid metabolism to full function. It takes about a year to build up fatty-tissue LA levels on a high-LA diet, so conquering overweight is a long-term project, with success infinitely more likely if an exercise programme is undertaken*.

## ARE YOU AN APPLE OR A PEAR?

Remember that insulin resistance (page 141) is associated with 'spare tyre' weight gain, and that this is a risk factor for diabetes, high blood pressure, heart attack, stroke and some forms of cancer. It seems that a fat tummy at least doubles your risk over that associated with other distribution of overweight.

You can discover where you fit in by measuring your waist (at 'the narrowest area above the umbilicus [navel]') and dividing by the hip measurement ('at the maximum gluteal [bottom] protrusion'). The table below is for ages 40-49, and exaggerates risks slightly if you're younger[148].

RISK AND WAIST-TO-HIP RATIO

| WAIST / HIPS | MALES | FEMALES |
|---|---|---|
| | Very High | |
| 1.0 | High | |
| | Moderate | |
| 0.9 | Low | Very High |
| | | High |
| 0.8 | " | Moderate |
| | | Low |
| 0.7 | " | |

*See also High Blood Pressure, page 174.

Exercise and the *Food for Vitality* eating pattern should lessen insulin resistance and tend to improve your waist-to-hip ratio.

## *Rheumatoid Arthritis*

This inflammatory form of rheumatism mainly affects those over 65, but about 5% of the population will suffer from it at some age. Rheumatoid arthritis is at least three thousand years old[149]* and can be crippling. It is thought to be an auto-immune disease, although its cause is unknown.

Conventional treatment consists of steroids or 'non-steroidal anti-inflammatories' (NSAIDs) like aspirin, phenacetin or acetaminophen for pain relief. These work by preventing inflammatory 2-series prostaglandin and thromboxane formation. Unfortunately, they also prevent the conversion of DGLA into beneficial, healing PGE1, so that both steroids and NSAIDs may actually have the long-term effect of *worsening* the disease[150]**.

A more natural approach is to manipulate dietary essential fatty acids to damp down the immune system, lessen production of inflammatory substances and boost PGE1.

When *Efamol* (12 capsules) and *Efamol Marine* (equivalent to 11 capsules of *Efamol* plus 240 mgs of EPA) was given to two groups of arthritics for a year, *60% of each group were able to give up their NSAID pain pills altogether* (although there was no evidence that the disease process itself was affected)[151]. Twenty-five per cent of the remaining *Efamol* group halved their doses of NSAIDs, as did 35% of the *Efamol Marine* group, but *both groups relapsed within three months of switching to placebos.*

Earlier studies used lesser quantities of evening primrose oil with lesser effects. *It seems certain that the **Food for Vitality***

*The Rheumatoid Arthritic pattern of bone loss was verified with X-rays in the remains of six persons who lived by the Tennessee River in north western Alabama between three and five thousand years ago.

**Of 112 participants, 54 were either dead (33%) or severely disabled (19%) after 20 years. Despite full treatment with steroids, gold and chloroquine, only 18% were leading a normal life (D. Scott et al., 'Long-Term Outcome of Treating Rheumatoid Arthritis: Results After 20 Years', *Lancet*, 16 May 1987, pp. 1108-1110).

*programme will benefit rheumatoid arthritics.* See also Food Allergy (page 151).

# Pregnancy

Any who contemplate parenthood should join Foresight, the Association for Pre-Conceptual Care* and buy their book *Planning for a Healthy Baby***. This organization has done a great deal to elucidate the causes of birth defects, infertility and prematurity. Their programme of testing and correcting vitamin, mineral and heavy metal levels is unique, innovative and effective. Entirely supported by subscription and voluntary efforts, their achievements are magnificent and inspiring.

The Foresight programme is available through doctors throughout the country. Inexpensive and easy to implement, it frequently solves infertility and turns out healthy babies much more reliably than standard medical care.

## EFAs in Pregnancy

The baby's brain and nervous system are bound to benefit from the pattern of eating advocated herein***. You can't make bricks without straw.

Several studies have shown that multivitamins lessen the incidence of neural tube defects, which are hideously unpleasant birth abnormalities[152]. Others indicate that the child's intelligence will be increased by supplementation[153] and by reducing refined

*The Old Vicarage, Church Lane, Witley, Godalming, Surrey GU8 5PN. Tel. (042879) 4500

**Belinda Barnes and Suzanne Bradley, *Planning for a Healthy Baby*, Ebury Press, London, 1990. Available from Murlyn Services Ltd., PO Box 50, Harlow, Essex CM17 0DZ, Tel. (0279) 427203.

***Dr William Connor of Oregon Health Sciences University has established that omega-3 deficient diets during pregnancy result in lowered visual acuity and, oddly enough, increased thirst in monkeys. He concluded that omega-3 fatty acid nutrition during both pregnancy and infancy must be considered of great importance to normal development in primates (W. Connor et al, 'Essentiality of n-3 Fatty acids: Evidence from the Primate Model', Program Abstracts, International Conference on the Health Effects of Omega-3 Polyunsaturated Fatty Acids, Washington DC, 1990).

foods and additives[154]. There's even evidence suggesting that immune system competence depends on adequate zinc during pregnancy – when mice mothers were deprived, their offspring had depressed immune function in spite of a normal diet, *and this effect persisted for two more generations*[155,156].

## Pre-Eclampsia: High Blood Pressure In Pregnancy

Between 5% and 7% of pregnant women develop very high blood pressure with swollen ankles and protein in the urine after six months of pregnancy. These women are likely to have decreased prostacyclin, the artery-dilating and blood-pressure-lowering prostaglandin, and there is now a sophisticated urine test* which can identify those at risk[157]. Since prostacyclin is an essential fatty acid derivative, *it is clearly important to keep the EFA-to-prostaglandin pathway in tip-top shape during pregnancy.*

## Post-Partum Depression

Interestingly, post-partum depression tends to happen in those who get PMS, and in those who breast-feed[158]. The essential fatty acids (EFAs) are known to be low in PMT, and there is a terrific drain on EFA reserves during breast-feeding. Therefore, it seems likely that post-partum depression may be *caused* by the consequent low PGE1, *and therefore relieved by GLA supplementation.*

## Prematurity

There's a link between magnesium and the ability to carry a baby to term which is so strong that '*failure to take magnesium supplements*' is actually considered a risk-factor for prematurity in West Germany. Some 10% of infants are born prematurely in the USA.

*The test looks for '2,3-dinor-6-keto-PGF1a', prostacyclin's breakdown product. In a normal pregnancy, this goes up by eight times, but in those who are likely to develop pre-eclampsia, the rise is only about three times.

## Foetal Alcohol Syndrome

Zinc deficiency and alcohol act synergistically to produce foetal alcohol syndrome, an appalling and unnecessary waste of life. The child of an alcoholic mother is likely to have characteristic facial deformities (eyes very wide apart and so forth), be retarded and experience profound behavioural difficulties. *In pregnant rats, evening primrose oil prevented much of this damage.*

Practically speaking, this means *anyone who drinks during pregnancy should take at least one capsule of evening primrose oil per drink*, although it is undoubtedly better to abstain completely.

## Again, Join Foresight

I could go on, but it's clear that the outcome of pregnancy is too important to leave to chance. Join the Foresight organization and undergo the Foresight screening at least a year before you intend to become pregnant, and *follow the* **Food for Vitality** *programme to nourish both of you properly.*

# *Premenstrual Tension*

The common symptoms of irritability, depression, breast pain, bloating, headaches and mood swings must occur within 14 days of, and clear up with, the menstrual period to be diagnosed as PMT. Eighty per cent of women suffer from it at some time in their lives, 10% very badly indeed.

A good book on this subject is Maryon Stewart's updated *Beat PMT Through Diet**. There is a section by Dr Guy Abraham, inventor of the *Optivite* supplement, an excellent overview and a clear review of the medical literature. Maryon Stewart and others started The Women's Nutritional Advisory Service**, which collects and disseminates information about PMT.

*Ebury Press, London, 1990
**PO Box 268, Hove, East Sussex, BN3 1RW. Tel. (0273) 771366

## BREAST DISEASE

Cyclical mastalgia means breast pain which is worse around the period, and this form of benign breast disease is helped by evening primrose oil in about 45% of cases. Plain mastalgia is helped somewhat, with about 27% responding[159]. However, only 6 *Efamol* capsules a day were used. A higher dose combined with fish in the diet and supplements of the vitamins and minerals needed by the EFA-to-prostaglandin pathway may be more effective.

Cystic breast disease – lumpy breasts – is relatively unresponsive to *Efamol*, but does improve when coffee is withdrawn.

# *Conclusion*

Despite all the scientific progress of the last 100 years, we have bungled badly when it comes to our diet. Perhaps we should have been more suspicious of food refining after the milling of grains was found to cause the deficiency disease beriberi, which probably killed millions of people. But food refining adds shelf life, increases appetite and therefore boosts consumption, and these economic advantages have proved too strong for our common sense.

Refined fats and hydrogenation emerged from food technologists' laboratories more than 80 years ago, but it's only recently become clear that they are partially responsible for the epidemic of Western degenerative diseases from which we suffer and die.

This book has attempted to steer a way out of this mess with a way of eating which meets our true requirements. We need essential fatty acids to preserve health, but other fats are mostly health-destroyers in any quantity. The next hurdle consists of getting enough of the co-nutrients such as vitamin C, vitamin $B_6$, vitamin $B_3$, zinc and magnesium which support essential oil use in the body. Then we must avoid the blockers of the essential fatty acid metabolism like saturated fat, margarine and high cholesterol. Finally, exercise seems to be necessary to get everything working properly.

Too complicated? *A diet of minimally processed natural foods provides all this* (*except the exercise*), and should finally 'result in the disappearance of the vast bulk of disease, misery and death' as Dr William Lane proposed so many decades ago. Other diseases will probably emerge from our poisoning of the environment, but *we can protect ourselves against the diseases we are familiar with – if we so choose.*

## The Changes To Come

Our children will face considerable challenges. Today, for every Westerner, there are three third-worlders aspiring to our wasteful ways, and some estimate the world population will eventually nearly *triple*[160]. Before long, the forests may be gone, the deserts spreading rapidly* and the oil which makes our high standard of living possible will certainly be running out. The pollution problem, which we haven't even begun to tackle, may be quite intrusive by then.

We're using irreplaceable natural resources to make goods *designed* to wear out, such as disposable nappies. However convenient such things may be, I can't help feeling that our descendants will not thank us for such poor stewardship of irreplaceable resources. The true cost of a disposable nappy may prove to be many hundreds of pounds when the cost to the environment is included.

Despite all this, *almost nobody advocates population control.* Perhaps our regard for the sanctity of human life somehow blinds us to the inevitable overcrowding, environmental destruction and massive die-back we can anticipate**. How ironic that our

*Remember that *the great deserts are man-made.* Chaco Canyon in New Mexico, a typical south western US desert area, was forested 1,800 years ago before the Anasazi Indians cut the trees down for fuel and building materials. Fossilized pollens show that Easter Island was forested before the Polynesians arrived and carved their statues – and deforested the island in less than four hundred years. The Mayan civilization probably did the same thing in Central America over a period of two thousand years (M. Kiefer, 'Fall of the Garden of Eden', *International Wildlife*, 1988), and the Sahara desert is supposed to have started with the felling of the cedars of Lebanon. *And it is chilling to reflect that standard American farming practice will cause the loss of all the topsoil within 50 years* ('Keeping Topsoil Down On The Farm', *Science News*, 1987, 132(23):357).

**John Malthus predicted this fate for humanity because he saw that it always occurred in animal populations which escaped environmental curbs.

unthinking regard for the sanctity of human life may result in its extinction.

However, these are wider issues, and the only things we can really control are personal. We are free to eat what we please (if we choose to overcome our addictions to unsuitable foods), and I am sure that the way of eating described in this book improves psychological health as well as physical health. Our children will inherit our mistakes, and the mistakes of generations before us, but by being all we can be, perhaps we can give them strength enough to face the challenges of survival.

# *Glossary of Terms*

**Antioxidants** are vitamins such as C and E, or enzymes such as glutathione peroxidase (which requires selenium to work) which neutralize free radicals, preventing destructive 'forest fire' self-propagating reactions in cell membranes etc. The body maintains an intricate and interdependent defence system of antioxidants.

**Arachidonic acid, AA,** 20:4w6 = 20 carbons, 4 double bonds. Omega-6 derivative of DGLA produced (mainly) in the liver or gained from meat, eggs or milk. Prominent component of cell membranes and about two-thirds of the omega-6 content of brain tissue. Important PGs derived from AA include PGI2 (prostacyclin) which lubricates arterial walls and PGE2 which is made by platelets and causes vasoconstriction and platelet aggregation. 2-series Thromboxanes and Leukotrienes made from AA mediate inflammation and chemotaxis (attract white cells to injuries). Paradoxically, when AA is *low*, larger quantities of undesirable PGs are made.

**Arteriosclerosis** or hardening of the arteries occurs when calcium is deposited in atherosclerotic plaque, making the arteries more rigid. The reason for the calcium deposits are unknown, but may be related to low magnesium and trace-mineral levels.

**Atherosclerosis** is the depositing of cholesterol and fat-containing plaque in the lining of the arteries.

**Beriberi** is the thiamin (vitamin $B_1$) deficiency disease which decimated the Orient when brown rice began to be milled. In dry beriberi, there is nerve deterioration and muscle wasting with paralysis and sometimes psychosis. In the wet form, fluids are trapped in the body so that the victim swells until death from congestive heart failure. These symptoms mimic those of many other diseases.

**Beta-carotene** is found in coloured vegetables such as carrots and dark green leaves. Also called pro-vitamin A because it consists of two vitamin A molecules, a storage form easily broken down to vitamin A as needed in the body. Functions as an antioxidant, protecting skin and mucous membranes, and is apparently highly protective against cancer. May protect skin against ultra-violet radiation since one of its functions in plants is to protect the delicate chlorophyll from ultra-violet light.

**Brown fat** gets its colour from large numbers of mitochondria, the tiny cellular fireplaces which burn glucose and fatty acids for energy to power cells. Brown fat cushions the back and neck and some vital organs, and can produce heat to maintain body temperature and/or burn off excess calories when instructed, perhaps by prostaglandins. Obesity may be related to poor brown fat performance.

**Carpal tunnel syndrome** occurs when inflammation of the wrist tendon running through the carpal tunnel to the fingers compresses nerves which also pass through the carpal tunnel. Although surgery is often used to relieve the pressure with varying success, carpal tunnel syndrome almost always responds to vitamin B6 supplementation *if the dose is large enough*.

**Cholesterol** is a steroid fat found in animal foods and also made in the body for hormones, vitamin D, cell wall and bile production. Cholesterol cannot be burned for calories in the body, and is an inert, waxy substance like candle wax. Cholesterol production in the liver appears to get out of control when the prostaglandins are disordered.

**cis- oils**: 'cis' means 'on the right side' and refers to double bonds between carbon atoms whose hydrogen atoms are on the same side of the carbon skeleton. Since hydrogen atoms repel each other, the carbon skeleton is bent. This means the melting point of the oil will be lower, and that the electrons in the crook of the bend in the skeleton form a 'pi-electron cloud' available for other functions, including roles in oxidative respiration.

**Cyclo-oxygenase** is the first enzyme to act on free fatty acids in their conversion to prostaglandins. Many drugs depend for their effect on inhibiting cyclo-oxygenase or preventing free fatty acids from reaching it. For example, steroid drugs inhibit release of free fatty acids, while aspirin-type drugs inhibit cyclo-oxygenase directly. Since arachidonic acid (AA) is the main PG precursor in most individuals subsisting on a land-based (Western) diet, and AA-derived prostaglandins are mostly inflammatory, steroids and aspirin-type drugs are effective against inflammation.

**DGLA, di-homo-gamma-linolenic acid,** 20:3w6 = 20 carbon atoms, three double bonds. This omega-6 derivative of linoleic acid is the immediate precursor of prostaglandin E1.

**Docosahexanoic acid, DHA,** 22:6w3 = 22 carbon atoms, 6 double bonds. Omega-3 derivative of (and storage form for) EPA, found in cold-water fish. Constitutes half of the fats in the brain.

**Double bond:** A bond is formed when two atoms share an electron, and a double bond involves two electrons. Double bonds occur between carbon atoms in the skeletons of fatty acids.

**EFA metabolism blockers** such as saturated fat, cholesterol, viruses, trans fats, excess glucose and ionizing radiation interfere with the 'delicate first step' delta-6-desaturase enzyme in the EFA pathway. This enzyme converts LA to GLA, and a working pathway is therefore essential for PGE1 production. Since PGE1 has many vital functions including control of other, less desirable prostaglandins, low PGE1 is associated with disease. Other blockers include deficiencies of insulin, vitamins B3, B6, C and the minerals zinc and magnesium.

**Essential fatty acids, EFAs,** are oils vital for health because the body cannot make them, so that they must be obtained from food. Their functions in the body include cell wall structure, cholesterol transport and serving as precursors of the prostaglandins, although they are also burned for calories.

**Free radical:** An electrically charged and therefore highly reactive atom or molecule such as the ozone ($O_3$) found in air pollution and cigarette smoke. About 5% of the oxygen we breathe ends up as free radicals, by-products of cellular energy production in the mitochondria (cellular energy producers), and must be neutralized by antioxidants such as SOD (superoxide dismutase) and vitamin E. Free radicals are also generated during the detoxification of toxins (for example, the headache remedy acetaminophen is seen by the body as a toxic substance) in the liver, during inflammation and by the immune system which uses 'respiratory bursts' of free radicals to damage the cell walls of invaders. If free radicals get out of control, they damage cells and organs – skin wrinkles and age spots are examples of out-of-control free radical activity.

**Gamma-linolenic acid, GLA,** 18:3w6 = 18 carbon atoms, 3 double bonds. The first EFA derivative made in the body from essential linoleic acid the 'delicate first step' enzyme, needed for both arachidonic acid and prostaglandin E1 production. The few dietary sources include human breast milk, evening primrose, borage and blackcurrant seed oils.

**High density lipoprotein, HDL:** transports fats from tissues to the liver. Contains cholesterol, but may scavenge cholesterol from plaque in the arterial lining. Formed when low density lipoprotein (LDL) gives up fats to tissues, a high level of HDL is protective against heart disease.

**Hormones** such as testosterone, thyroxin, growth hormone and adrenalin are made in the endocrine (ductless) glands (testes, thyroid, pituitary, adrenals etc.), distributed in the blood and affect numerous metabolic and growth functions. Contrast Prostaglandin.

**Hydrogenated fat:** an unsaturated oil forced to combine with hydrogen by high temperatures and catalysts. Margarine and shortening contain abundant hydrogenates. Partially hydrogenated essential fats fail to function as EFAs in the body, and actually increase EFA requirements. This interference in the EFA-to-prostaglandin pathway may be the final insult which precipitates heart attacks.

**Leukotrienes, LTs.** When free fatty acids are acted upon by lipoxygenase instead of cyclo-oxygenase, leukotrienes are formed. Lipoxygenase is present in the skin of patients with psoriasis, and LTs can induce bronchial constriction (as in asthma) and leakage of the microvasculature, indicating that they have a role in the allergic response. Other LTs are made by immune system white cells and induce other cells to congregate.

**Linoleic acid, LA,** 18:2w6 = 18 carbon atoms, 2 double bonds. The omega-6 essential fatty acid which cannot be made in the body and which must be obtained from seeds, nuts etc., where it is more plentiful in cold-adapted species. Dietary levels are usually 7–10%, which would be adequate but for the presence of trans forms and EFA metabolism blockers such as saturated fat. Plentiful LA in body fat appears protective against overweight, high blood pressure and heart disease, although this protection is mediated through the prostaglandin metabolism so a functioning EFA-to-PG pathway is needed.

**Linolenic acid, LNA,** 18:3w3 = 18 carbons, 3 double bonds. Essential omega-3 fatty acid which cannot be made in the body. Made by marine plants and animals, and also by cold-adapted northern species of nuts, grains and seeds. Flaxseed oil is 57% of LNA, which is converted into EPA and DHA in the body. Also known as Alpha-linolenic acid.

**Lipoxygenase** is an enzyme which acts on the free fatty acids to produce leukotrienes, which are part of the allergic response. These highly inflammatory substances are undesirable except when necessary to fight infection or in trauma.

**Low density lipoprotein, LDL:** made in the liver, this fat, protein and cholesterol package transports fatty acids and cholesterol from the liver to tissues in need of them. LDL production seems to be controlled by prostaglandins, so that when prostaglandin formation is disturbed by, for example, excess fat intake LDL cholesterol rises. High LDL is a marker for high risk of heart disease.

**Mono-unsaturates** are oils with one double bond. The best known is oleic acid (18:1w9) which is found in olive oil. Since oleic acid is stable under heating, olive oil is a better choice for cooking than polyunsaturated oils.

**Obesity** is often defined as body weight 20% or more above normal.

**Omega** notation for fatty acids. 18:2w6 is the omega notation for linoleic acid and tells us that it contains 18 carbon atoms with 2 double bonds. The number following the w is the number of carbon atoms from the end of the molecule before the first double bond. This completely defines fatty acids with natural or cis bonds because these are always 'methylene-interrupted', meaning their double bonds are always separated by a carbon atom.

**Pellagra** is the niacin (vitamin B3) deficiency disease which was endemic in the industrialized world after the turn of the century. The four Ds of pellagra stand for diarrhoea, dermatitis, dementia and death. Insane asylums were filled with pellagra victims. Worst hit were American sharecropping families living on corn, lard and white flour *although traditional eaters such as South American Indian tribes obtain vitamin B3 from corn by treatment with lime.*

**Placebo**: a dummy medication given in scientific experiments to discover how much expectation influences outcome.

**Pottenger's Effect** is the progressive deterioration over several generations seen in people (and cats) eating diets which do not fulfil their requirements. There are allergic manifestations, narrowed dental arches, irritability and poor skin (fur) which become worse with each passing generation.

**Prostaglandins Pgs**: A group of hormone-like substances made from the essential fatty acids in tissues to control a bewildering number of local conditions, including platelet aggregation (a first step in blood clotting), lubrication of the arterial wall and blood vessel constriction or dilation. Their lives are much shorter than those of hormones and most are destroyed in their first pass through the lungs, if not before.

**Prostaglandin E1, PGE1**: a desirable prostaglandin whose effects include regulation of cholesterol production in the liver, dilation of the blood vessels and immune system control (which combats allergic reactions and immune system over-reaction as in arthritis). For adequate PGE1 production, a diet containing the essential fatty acids and their co-factors such as vitamins C, B6, B3, magnesium and zinc is needed. Too much of Pottenger's effect (q.v.), ageing or viral infection may mean evening primrose oil supplementation is required to fulfil PGE1 production.

**Prostate gland**: encircles the urethra below the bladder in the male and supplies prostaglandins to the seminal fluid which may suppress immune reactions against spermatozoa in the female. These prostaglandins are plentiful, and since they were the first to be discovered and were then thought to be unique to the prostate, prostaglandins were named for the gland.

**Saturated fats** have no double bonds, and therefore no potential for accepting more hydrogen atoms. They tend to be more solid than unsaturates. Rare in nature, they are artifacts of intensive rearing practices in agriculture designed to achieve maximum weight gain with minimum food input. Unfortunately, they are catastrophically bad for health.

**Thromboxanes, TXs** are, like the leukotrienes (q.v.), inflammatory essential fatty acid derivatives which aggregate the platelets and constrict the blood vessels.

**trans- fats** are usually the result of hydrogenation, although some are formed in the rumens of grazing animals and therefore appear naturally in dairy products. 'trans' means 'on the other side' and refers to an unnatural double bond between carbon atoms whose hydrogen atoms are on opposite sides of the carbon skeleton. This is unfortunate because the molecule is straighter and behaves more like a saturated fat. Although this is not a problem when the fatty acid is burned for energy, it becomes a very real problem in the essential fatty acid metabolism because trans fats tie up the enzymes and block the pathway for a time. This increases essential fatty acid requirements, often beyond the available supply.

# *Further Reading*


Belinda Barnes and Irene Colquhoun, *The Hyperactive Child*, Thorsons, Wellingborough, Northamptonshire, 1984.

Charles Bates, Ph.D., *Essential Fatty Acids in Immunity and Mental Health*, Life Sciences Press, Tacoma WA, 1987, Tel. (206) 922-0442

Beata Bishop, *A Time to Heal*, Severn House Publishers, 1985

Robert Buist, *Food Intolerance*, Prism Press, Sherborne, Dorset, 1984.

Michael Crawford, MD, and David Marsh, *The Driving Force*, William Heinemann Ltd., London, UK, 1989

Udo Erasmus, *Fats and Oils*, Alive Books, Vancouver, Canada, 1986

Ben Feingold, MD, *Why your Child is Hyperactive*, Random House, New York, 1974

Max Gerson, MD, *A Cancer Therapy: Results of Fifty Cases*. Totality Books, Del Mar, California, 1958. Available from the Gerson Institute, PO Box 430, 5012 Central Avenue #E, Bonita, CA 92002, USA, Tel. (619) 267-1150.

Anne Louise Gittleman, *Beyond Pritikin*, Bantam, London, 1988

Judy Graham, *Multiple Sclerosis, A Self-Help Guide to Its Management*, Healing Arts Press, Rochester, Vermont, USA, 1989

Arthur Janov, Ph.D., *The New Primal Scream*, Abacus, London, 1991

Dr Alan Levin and Merla Zellerbach, *The Type 1/Type 2 Allergy Relief Program*, Berkeley, New York, 1983

John Ott, *Health and Light*, Pocket Books, New York, 1973

Linus Pauling, *How to Live Longer and Feel Better*, W.H. Freeman and Company, New York, 1986

Francis M. Pottenger, Jr, MD, *Pottenger's Cats: A Study in Nutrition*. Price-Pottenger Nutrition Foundation, 1983, see below for order information.

Weston A. Price, DDS, *Nutrition and Physical Degeneration: A Comparison of Primitive and Modern Diets and Their Effects*. Price-Pottenger Nutrition Foundation, 1982; still available from P.P.N.F, PO Box 2614, La Mesa, CA 92044-2614, USA, Tel. (714) 582 4168.

Theron Randolph and Ralph Moss, *An Alternative Approach to Allergies*, Harper and Row, New York, 1980

Maryon Stewart, *Beat PMT Through Diet*, Ebury Press, London, 1990

# *Organizations Worthy of Your Support*

Become a member of the Price-Pottenger Nutrition Foundation – you get the P.P.N.F Journal (which gives unbiased information on new books, the environment, holistic pet care, natural therapies etc.), nutritional advice for the asking, referrals to an international network of holistic health professionals, and, most important of all, you support a group dedicated to the principle that the quality of our soil and the health and well-being of our planet and animal kingdoms determine the physical foundations of human life, which in turn promotes balanced mental and spiritual being. Price-Pottenger Nutrition Foundation, PO Box 2614, La Mesa, CA 92044-2614, USA. Tel. (714) 5821 4168.

Subscribe to the Gerson Foundation Healing Newsletter, $20/year outside the US, for a critical review of developments in the cancer industry, up-to-the-minute summaries of holistic cancer therapy research and a fascinating perspective on developments in the health field. Highly recommended. The Gerson Institute, PO Box 430, 5012 Central Avenue #E, Bonita, CA 92002, USA, Tel. (619) 267-1150.

The Hyperactive Children's Support Group, 71 Whyke Lane, Chichester, West Sussex PO19 2LD.

Foresight, The Association for Pre-Conceptual Care, The Old Vicarage, Church Lane, Witley, Godalming, Surrey GU8 5PN. Tel. (042879) 4500 between 9.30 a.m. and 7.30 p.m.

The Women's Nutritional Advisory Service, PO Box 268, Hove, East Sussex, BN3 1RW. Tel. (0273) 771366. The W.N.A.S. collects and disseminates information on PMT.

# *Sources*

Bioceuticals Limited (Linseed Oil), 26 Zennor Road, London SW12 0PS. Tel. (081) 675-5664, make and distribute edible flaxseed (linseed) oil.

Nutricology Inc., 400 Preda Street, San Leandro, CA 94577-0489

– Tel. (415) 639-4572. Nutricology can supply many of the products mentioned in this book through the post, including Chronoset (a source of melatonin – see page 149).

*Optivite* is distributed by Booker Nutritional Products, Beaver House, Byfleet, Surrey KT14 7HN

*Efamol* is manufactured by Efamol Ltd., and distributed by Brittania Health Products, Forum House, 41–51 Brighton Road, Redhill, Surrey RH1 6YS

I have no commercial association with any of these companies.

# *References*

## INTRODUCTION

1. 'The Heart of Depression', *Science News*, 135(1):13, 1989
2. 'Hostility Boosts Risk of Heart Trouble', *Science News*, 135(4):60, 1989

## CHAPTER 1: LIVE LONG AND PROSPER

1. 'Depression and Cancer: A Fatal Link', *Science News*, 132(16):244 (1987). 'The finding that depression is associated more strongly with cancer mortality than with cancer incidence suggests it may promote rather than initiate the disease process.'
2. This is an observation of the Hyperactive Children's Support Group, 71 Whyke Lane, Chichester, West Sussex, PO19 2LD
3. S.E. Strauss et al., 'Allergy and the Chronic Fatigue Syndrome', *J. Allergy and Clinical Immunology*, 81:791-95 (1988)
4. A. Atton-Chamla et al., 'Premenstrual Syndrome and Atopy', *Pharmatherapeutica*, 2(7):481-486 (1980)
5. M.S. Manku et al., 'Reduced Levels of Prostaglandin Precursors in the Blood of Atopic Patients: Defective Delta-6-Desaturase Function as a Biological Basis for Atopy', *Prostaglandins, Leukotrienes and Medicine*, 9:615-628 (1982)
6. P. Hoffman et al., 'Enhancement of the Anti-Hypertensive Effect of Dietary n3 and n6-PUFA in SHR During a Four-Generation Feeding Period', *Biomed. Biochim. Acta*, 43(8/9):S277-S230 (1984)
7. 'No-Fault Fat: More Praise For Fish Oil', *Science News*, 134(15):228 (1988)
8. P. Hoffman et al., 'Enhancement of the Anti-Hypertensive Effect of Dietary n3 and n6-PUFA in SHR During a Four-Generation Feeding Period', *Biomed. Biochim. Acta*, 43(8/9):S227-S230 (1984)
9. A.J. Houtsmuller et al., 'Favourable Influences of Linoleic Acid on the Progression of Diabetic Micro-and Macroangiopathy in Adult Onset Diabetes Mellitus', *Prog. Lipids Research*, 20:377-386 (1982)

# Chapter 2: What to Eat


1. A. Sanchez et al., 'Role of Sugars in Human Neutrophilic Phagocytosis', *Am. J. Clin. Nutr.*, 26:1180- 1184 (1973)
2. Dozens of studies hint at this, such as Pudelkewicz, C., et al., 'Requirements of the Female Rat for Linoleic And Linolenic Acids', *J. Nutr.*, 1968, 64:138
3. M. Sugano et al., 'Hypocholesterolemic Effect of Gamma-Linolenic Acid as Evening Primrose Oil', *Ann. Nutr. Metab.*, 30:289-299 (1986)
4. D. Horrobin, 'The Lowering of Plasma Cholesterol by Essential Fatty Acids', in D. Horrobin, ed., *Clinical Uses of the Essential Fatty Acids*, Eden Press, Canada, 1982
5. Linus Pauling, *How to Live Longer and Feel Better*, W.H. Freeman, New York, 1986, p.240
6. C. Krogh, ed., *Compendium of Pharmaceuticals and Specialties*. Canadian Pharmaceutical Association, Ottawa, 1983
7. J.P. Carter, 'Gamma-Linolenic Acid as Nutrient', *Food Technology*, June, 1988
8. K. West, 'Diet Therapy for Diabetes: An Analysis of Failure', *Annals of Internal Medicine*, 79:425-434 (1973)
9. R. Mensink et al., 'Effect of Dietary Trans Fatty Acids on High-Density and Low-Density Lipoprotein Cholesterol Levels in Healthy Subjects', *New England Journal of Medicine*, 323(7):439-455 (1990)
10. L. Thomas et al., 'Concentration of transunsaturated Fatty Acids in the Adipose Tissue of Decedents Dying of Ischaemic Heart Disease Compared with Controls', *J. Epidemiology and Community Health*, 37:22-24 (1983)
11. R. Rizek et al., 'Symposium: Status of Fat in Food and Nutrition', *Journal of the American Oil Chemists' Society*, 51:244-250 (1974)
12. F. Mattson et al., 'Effect of Hydrogenated Fat on the Plasma Cholesterol and Triglyceride Level of Man', *The Americal Journal of Clinical Nutrition*, 28:726-731, (1975)
13. P. Oster et al., 'Blood Pressure and Adipose Tissue Linoleic Acid', *Res. Exp. Med.*, 175:287-291 (1979); P. Oster et al., 'Linoleic Acid and Blood Pressure', *Prog. Fd. Nutr. Sci.*, 4(5):39-40 (1980)
14. R. Lowndes et al., 'The Effects of Evening Primrose Oil Administration on the Serum Lipids of Normal and Obese Human Subjects', in D. Horrobin, ed., *Clinical Uses Of The Essential Fatty Acids*, Eden Press, Canada, 1982.
15. A.E. Hansen, 'Role of Unsaturated Dietary Fat in Infant Nutrition', *Am. J. Pub. Health*, 47:1367-1370 (1957); A.E. Hansen et al., 'Essential Fatty Acids in Human Nutrition', *J. Nutr.*, 60:565-576 (1958)
16. J. Douglass et al., 'Obesity Regimen', *Medical Tribune*, 25:30, 25 January 1984; J. Douglass et al., 'Effects of a Raw Food Diet on Hypertension and Obesity', *Southern Medical Journal*, 78(7):841-844 (1985)
17. G. Abraham, 'The Calcium Controversy', *J. Applied Nutrition*, 34(2):69-73
18. 'New Misgivings About Low Magnesium', *Science News*, 133(23):356 (1988)
19. J. Perera, 'The Hazards of Heavy Breathing', *New Scientist*, 120(641):46-48
20. D. Polley et al., 'Dietary Vitamin $B_6$ in College Students', Nutrition Reports

International, 31(2)281-285 (1985); E. Pao et el., 'Problem Nutrients in the United States', *Food Technology*, pp. 58-69 (September 1981)
21. 'Possible Vitamin $B_6$ Deficiency Uncovered in Persons with the "Chinese Restaurant Syndrome" ', *Nutrition Reviews*, 40(1):15-16 (1982)
22. J.R. Beetens et al., 'Influence of Vitamin C on the Metabolism of Arachidonic Acid and the Development of Aortic Lesions during Experimental Atherosclerosis in Rabbits', *Biochem. Biochim. Acta* 43:S274-S276 (1984)
23. S. Levine et al., *Antioxidant Adaptation And Its Role In Free Radical Pathology*, Biocurrents, San Leandro, 1985
24. 'Vitamin C – Were the Trials Well Controlled and Are Large Doses Safe', *Medical Letter*, 28 May 1971
25. D. Eddy and D. Harman, 'Free Radical Theory of Aging: Effect of Age, Sex and Dietary Precursors on Rat Brain Docosahexanoic Acid', *J. American Geriatrics Society*, 25(5):428-437
26. David Horrobin, Personal Communication, 22 August 1989

## CHAPTER 3: EAT, DRINK AND BE WARY

1. Francis M. Pottenger, Jr., M.D., *Pottenger's Cats: A Study in Nutrition.* Price-Pottenger Nutrition Foundation, 1983
2. Weston A. Price, D.D.S., *Nutrition and Physical Degeneration: A Comparison of Primitive and Modern Diets and Their Effects.* Price-Pottenger Nutrition Foundation, 1982; still available from Price-Pottenger Nutrition Foundation, PO Box 2614, La Mesa, CA 92044-2614 USA. Tel. (714) 582 4168
3. C. Galli and A. Socini, 'Dietary Lipids in pre- and post-natal Development.' In *Dietary Fats and Health*, Pekins and Visek, eds., American Oil Chemists Society, (1983)
4. Dobbing, 1972, cited in M. Crawford and D. Marsh, *The Driving Force*, William Heinemann Ltd., UK (1989)
5. A. Sinclair and M. Crawford (1973), cited in M. Crawford and D. Marsh, *The Driving Force*, William Heinemann Ltd., UK (1989)
6. R.W. Smithels et al., 'Possible Prevention of Neural-Tube Defects by Preconceptual Vitamin Supplementation', *Lancet*, i:339 (1980)
7. D.J.P. Barker and C. Osmond, 'Inequalities in Health in Britain', *Lancet*, i:1077-81, 1986
8. G. Osborne, 'Stages in the Development of Coronary Disease Observed in 1500 Young Subjects', in *Editions du Centre National de la Recherche Scientifique*, Paris, 1967
9. Crawford & Hansen (1970), cited in M. Crawford and D. Marsh, *The Driving Force*. W. Heinemann Ltd., UK, 1989
10. J.J. McNamara et al., 'Coronary Artery Disease in Combat Casualties in Vietnam', *JAMA*, 216(7):1185-1187 (1971). 5% showed severe atherosclerosis, while 45% showed evidence of atherosclerosis.
11. H.M. Sinclair, 'Deficiency of Essential Fatty Acids and Atherosclerosis, etcetera', *Lancet*, April 7, 1956, pp. 381-83
12. W.E. and S.J. Connor, 'The Key Role of Nutritional Factors in the Prevention of Coronary Heart Disease', *Prev. Med.*, 1:49-83 (1972)

13. S. Wright, 'Essential Fatty Acids and Atopic Eczema: Biological and Immunological Studies' in *Omega-6 Essential Fatty Acids: Pathophysiology and Roles in Clinical Medicine*, ed. D. Horrobin, Wiley-Liss, NY, 1990
14. *Omega-6 Essential Fatty Acids: Pathophysiology and Roles in Clinical Medicine*, ed. David Horrobin, Wiley-Liss, NY, 1990.
15. Donald Rudin et al., *The Omega-3 Phenomenon*. Sidgwick and Jackson, London, 1988
16. 'Where levels of all D6D metabolites are down, the conversion of arachidonic acid to 2-series prostaglandins is consistently increased. [Probably] a fall in . . . cyclic AMP consequent upon reduced production of PGE1 from DGLA [allows] mobilization of arachidonic acid from phospholipid stores', (D. Horrobin, 'Regulation of Prostaglandin Biosynthesis by the Manipulation of Essential Fatty Acid Metabolism', *Rev. Pure and Appl. Pharm. Sci.*, 1983, 4:339-383).

## CHAPTER 4: GETTING BETTER

1. G.A. Jamal, 'Prevention and Treatment of Diabetic Distal Polyneuropathy by the Supplementation of Gamma-linolenic Acid', in *Omega-6 Essential Fatty Acids: Pathophysiology and Roles in Clinical Medicine*, ed. David Horrobin, Wiley-Liss, NY, 1990.
2. A.I.M. Glen et al., 'Essential Fatty Acids and Alcoholism', in D.F. Horrobin, ed., *Omega-6 Essential Fatty Acids*, Wiley Liss, New York NY, 1990
3. *Omega-6 Essential Fatty Acids: Pathophysiology and Roles in Clinical Medicine*, ed. David Horrobin, Wiley-Liss, NY, 1990
4. B. Jacobsen et al., 'Perinatal Origin of Adult Self-Destructive Behaviour', *Acta. Psyciatr. Scand.*, 76:364-371 (1987)
5. J.A. Wilcox and H.A. Nasrallah, 'Perinatal Distress and Prognosis of Psychotic Illness', *Biological Psychiatry*, 17:173-175 (1987)
6. B. Bower, 'Crossing the "Borderline" of Child Abuse', *Science News*, 135(16):246 (22 April 1989)
7. K. Fackelman, 'Brain and Immunity: Mapping the Link', *Science News*, 136(3):36, 1989
8. C. Vaughan, 'The Depression–Stress Link', *Science News*, 134(10):155,1988
9. A. Janov, *The Anatomy of Mental Illness*. Putnam's, NY, 1971
10. S. Boyd Eaton et al., *The Paleolithic Prescription*, Harper and Row, New York, 1988; Leon Chaitow, *The Stone Age Diet*, Macdonald & Co., London, 1987
11. Jo Durned-Smith and Diane de Simone, *Sex and the Brain*, Pan, London, 1983

## CHAPTER 5: DERANGED ESSENTIAL FATTY ACID DISEASES

1. H.M. Sinclair, 'Deficiencies of the Essential Fatty Acids and Atherosclerosis, Etcetera', *Lancet*, i:381-383 (1956); 'Sees Essential Fatty Acid Lack Causing Degenerative Disease', *4th Ann. Drug Trade Survey*, 3&7 (1957); 'Food

and Health', *Br. Med. J.*, 2:1424-1426 (1957); 'Essential Fatty Acids and Chronic Degenerative Diseases', in J. Rose, ed., *Nutrition and Killer Diseases*, NJ Noyes, 1982, pp. 69-83

2. D.F. Horrobin, 'Regulation of Prostaglandin Biosynthesis by the Manipulation of Essential Fatty Acid Metabolism', *Rev. Pure and Appl. Pharm. Sci.*, 4(4):340-383 (1983)
3. C. Bates, *Essential Fatty Acids and Immunity in Mental Health*. Life Sciences Press, Tacoma WA, 1987. Tel. (206) 272-0530
4. W. Insull et al., 'Studies of Arteriosclerosis in Japanese and American Men I', *J. Clin. Investigation*, 48:1313-1327 (1969)
5. P. Darcet et al., 'Effect of a Diet Enriched with GLA on PUFA Metabolism and Platelet Aggregation in Elderly Men', *Ann. Nutr. Al.*, 1980, 34:277-290
6. R.L. Walford, *Maximum Lifespan*, Avon, New York, 1983. R.L. Walford, *The 120-Year Diet*, Simon & Schuster, New York, 1986
7. F.H. Faas and W.J. Carter, 'Altered Fatty Acid Desaturation and Microsomal Fatty Acid Composition in the Streptozotocin Diabetic Rat', Lipids, 15:953-961 (1980)
8. 'Highballs and the Heart', *Science News*, 134(7):106 (1988)
9. D.F. Horrobin et al., 'Possible Role of Prostaglandin E1 in the Affective Disorders and in Alcoholism', *British Medical Journal*, 280(6228):1363-1366 (1980)
10. J. Graham, *Evening Primrose Oil*. Thorsons, Wellingborough, Northamptonshire, 1988
11. B. Seeman et al., 'Mimicry of Dopamine Stimulation of Hypothalamic Pathways in C3a Anaphylatoxin', *Soc. Neurosci. Abstr.*, 1310:414 (1978)
12. C. Bates, *Essential Fatty Acids and Immunity in Mental Health*. Life Sciences Press, Tacoma WA, 1987. Tel. (206) 272-0530
13. 'A Problem of Definition', *Science News*, 134(5):75
14. A. Glen et al., 'Essential Fatty Acids and Alcoholism', in D. Horrobin, ed., *Omega-6 Essential Fatty Acids*, Wiley-Liss, NY, 1990
15. R. Rizek, 'Fat in Today's Food Supply – Levels of Use and Sources', *J. Am. Oil Chemists' Soc.*, 51:244-250 (1974)
16. J. Budwig, *Die elementare Funktion der Atmung in ihrer Beziehung zu autoxydablen Nahrungstoffen*, Hyperion Verlag, Frieberg, W. Germany, 1956; *Oel-Eiweiss Kost*, Hyperion Verlag, 1955; *Krebs ein Fett-Probelm*, Hyperion Verlag, 1956; *Das Fettsyndrom*, Hyperion Verlag, 1959; *Kosmische Kraefte gegen Krebs*, Hyperion Verlag, 1966; *Laserstrahlen gegen Krebs*, Hyperion Verlag, 1968; *Fette als wahre Hilfe*, Hyperion Verlag, 1972; *Der Tod des Tumours*, Freudenstadt, 1977; *Der Tod des Tumours Band 2*, Freudenstadt, 1977; *Fotoelemente des Lebens*, Resch Verlag, Innsbruck, Austria, 1979; *Fettfibel*, 1979. Translations and imterpretations of her work have appeared in English: J. Budwig, 'The Photoelements of Life', *Search for Health APW News Bulletin*, PO Box 75337, St Paul, MN 55175, 2(2):11-13 (1988); Udo Erasmus, *Fats and Oils*, Alive Books, Vancouver, Canada, 1986; Dan C. Roehm, MD, 3450 Park Central Blvd. North, Pompano Beach, FL 33064, 'The Biologic Electron: Re-examining the Work of Johanna Budwig', *Townsend Letter for Doctors* (July, 1990):480-482. Roehm points out that any interested doctor can set up in an office laboratory to diagnose and monitor the progress of cancer patients

by the Budwig method, as described in 'Die elementare Funktion der Atmung . . .' cited above, and that he personally has satisfied himself by this means that her approach works as effectively as she declares.

17. Johanna Budwig, 'Die Papierchromatographie der Blutlipoide, Geschwulstproblem und Fettorschung – Neue Wege der Fettanalyse', in *Fette und Siefen*, Industrieverlag, Hamburg, 1950
18. Udo Erasmus, *Fats and Oils*. Alive Books, Vancouver, 1986, p. 274
19. M. Gerson, *A Cancer Therapy: Results of Fifty Cases*. Totality Books, Del Mar, California, 1958. Highly recommended, available from the Gerson Institute, 5012 Central Avenue #E, Bonita, CA 92002, USA. Tel. (619)267-1150. The journalist S.J. Haught set out to debunk Gerson as a quack (the American Medical Association position) and ended up writing *Cancer? Think Curable*! after interviewing his patients. Beata Bishop, an English melanoma patient cured at the Gerson facility in Mexico, wrote *A Time to Heal* (Severn House Publishers, 1985). These books are also available from the Gerson Institute. Gerson actually presented five cured cancer patients to a Senate sub-comittee investigating cancer and chaired by Claude Pepper in 1946. He failed to get research funds by just four votes after a massive medical lobbying effort.
20. *Gerson Healing Newsletter*, October 1984, Newsletter #3, p. 7
21. C.F. Van de Merwe et al., 'Oral Gamma-linolenic acid in 21 Patients with Untreatable Malignancy. An Ongoing Pilot Open Clinical Trial', *Brit. J. Clin Pract.*, 41(9):907-915 (1987)
22. L.M. Dunbar et al., 'Enzyme Deletions and EFA Metabolism in Cultured Cells', *J. Biol. Chem.*, 1975, 250:1152-54
23. 'Harnessing Fatty Acids to Fight Cancer', *Science News*, 133:332; M.E.Begin et al., 'Selective Killing of Human Cancer Cells by Polyunsaturated Fatty acids', *Prostaglandins Leukotrienes Med.*, 1985, 19:177-86
24. L.R. Bennet et al., 'Effects of Ultracentrifugal Fractions of Small Intestine Tissues Upon Transplanted Lymphosarcoma', *Proc. Soc. Exp. Biol. Med.*, 1951, 78:790-1; L.R. Bennet et al., 'Further Studies of a Small Intestine Microsomal Fraction Upon Transplantable Tumours', *Proc. Soc. Exp. Biol. Med.*, 1953, 82:665-8; L.R. Bennet et al., 'Effect of Lytic Agents on Plasma Membrane of Ehrlich Ascitic Tumour Cells and Mouse Erythrocytes', *JNCI*, 1957, 19:999-1011; J. Booyens et al., Some Effects of the Essential Fatty Acids . . . on the Proliferation of Human Osteogenic Sarcoma Cells in Culture', *Prostaglandins Leukotrienes Medicine*, 1984, 15:15-33; M.E. Begin et al., 'Differential Killing of Human Carcinoma Cells Supplemented with n3 and n6 Polyunsaturated Fatty Acids', *JNCI*, 1986, 77:1053-62; I. Siegal et al., 'Cytotoxic Effects of Free Fatty Acids on Ascites Tumour Cells', *JNCI*, 1987, 78:271-77; H. Yoshikawa et al., 'Potentiation of Antitumour Effect of Bleomycin by Lipid- Surfactant Mixed Micelles', *Pharm. Dynamics*, 1985, 8:143-151; 'Dietary Oils and Melanoma', *British Journal of Surgery*, June 1988
25. A. Norman et al., 'Antitumour Activity of Sodium Linoleate', Nutrition and Cancer, 1988, 11(2):107-15
26. I. Wickelgren, 'More Veggies Join Fight Against Lung Cancer', *Science News*, 136(7):102, 1989
27. S. Graham et al., 'Alimentary Factors in the Epidemiology of Gastric

Cancer', *Cancer*, 1972, 30:927-38; W. Haenszel et al., 'Stomach Cancer among Japanese in Hawaii', *J. Natl. Cancer Inst.*, 1972, 49:969-88; W. Haenszel et al., 'Stomach Cancer in Japan', *J. Natl. Cancer Inst.*, 1976, 56:265-74, etc. These studies were cited in the US National Research Council's *Diets, Nutrition, and Cancer* (National Academy Press, Washington, DC, 1982: Ch. 17 – 'The Relationship of Diet to Cancer at Specific Sites')

**28.** J. Raloff, 'Coming – Dietary Aids to Prevent Cancer?', *Science News*, 1987, 131(13):206

**29.** E. Cameron and L. Pauling, 'Supplemental Ascorbate in the Supportive Treatment of Cancer'. *Proceedings of the National Academy of Science*, I: 73:3685-3689 (1976); II: 75:6252-6256 (1979)

**30.** F. Morishige and A. Murata, 'Prolongation of Survival Times in Terminal Human Cancer by Administration of Supplemental Ascorbate', *Journal of the International Academy of Preventive Medicine*, 5:1-8, (1978)

**31.** E. Creagan, C. Moertel et al., 'Failure of High-Dose Vitamin C (Ascorbic Acid) Therapy to Benefit Patients With Advanced Cancer: A Controlled Trial', *New England Journal of Medicine*, 301:687-690 (1979)

**32.** C. Moertel et al., 'High-Dose Vitamin C versus Placebo In The Treatment Of Patients Who Have Had No Prior Chemotherapy', *New England Journal of Medicine*, 312(3):137-141 (1985)

**33.** C. Tsao et al., 'Evidence of Rebound Effect With Ascorbic Acid', *Medical Hypotheses*, 13:303-310 (1984)

**34.** E. Cameron and L Pauling, 'On Cancer and Vitamin C', *Executive Health*, 16(4):1-8 (1980)

**35.** M. Carpenter, 'Pauling Reminder: Vitamin C a Hallowed Wound-Healing Aid', *Medical Tribune*, 21939):6 (3 December 1980)

**36.** L. Williams et al., 'Serum Fatty Acid Proportions Are Altered During the Year Following Acute Epstein-Barr Virus Infection', *Lipids*, 23910):981-988

**37.** P. and W. Behan, 'Essential Fatty Acids in the Treatment of Postviral Fatigue Syndrome', in D. Horrobin, ed., *Omega-6 Essential Fatty Acids*, Wiley-Liss, NY, 1990

**38.** R. Cathcart, 'Vitamin C, Titrating to Bowel Tolerance, Anascorbemia, and Acute Induced Scurvy', *Medical Hypotheses*, 7:1359-1376 (1981)

**39.** C. Tsao et al., 'Evidence Of Rebound Effect With Ascorbic Acid', *Medical Hypotheses*, 13:303-310 (1984)

**40.** J. Graham, *Evening Primrose Oil*. Thorsons, Wellingborough, Northamptonshire, 1988

**41.** T. Merimee, 'Diabetic Retinopathy, A Synthesis of Perspectives', *New England Journal of Medicine*, 322(14):976-983 (1990)

**42.** Tateki Hayashi et al., 'Formation of the N,N'-Dialkylpyrazine Cation Radical from Glyoxal Dialkylimine Produced on Reaction of a Sugar with an Amine or Amino Acid', *Agric. Biol. Chem.*, 49(11):3131-3137 (1985).

**43.** 'Bulging Bellies and Breast Cancer', *Nutrition Action Newsletter*, 17(3):4 (April 1990).

**44.** 'Cold Facts on Diabetes', *Science News*, 134(8):117 (1988)

**45.** A. Houtsmuller, 'The Role of Fats in the Treatment of Diabetes Mellitus', in Vergroessen, *The Role of Fats in Human Nutrition*, Academic Press, London, 1975

46. 'Magnesium Eases Diabetic Blood Pressure', *Science News*. 138(12):189 (1990)
47. 'Reduced Levels of Magnesium Reported to Correlate with Diabetic Retinopathy', *Medical Tribune*, 21(39):2 (3 December 1980)
48. H. Shroeder et al., 'Chromium Deficiency as a Factor in Atherosclerosis', *J. Chron. Dis.* 23:123-142 (1970).
49. J. Douglass, 'Raw Diet and Insulin Requirements', *Annals of Internal Medicine*, 82(1):61-62 (1975); J. Douglass and I. Rasgon, 'Diet and Diabetes', *Lancet*, 11 December 1976, p. 1306
50. Albert Sanchez et al., 'Role of Sugars in Human Neutrophilic Phagocytosis', *The American Journal of Clinical Nutrition*, 1973, 26:1180-84.
51. P. Crapo et al., 'Comparison of Serus Glucose, Insulin and Glucagon Responses to Different Types of Complex Carbohydrage in Non-Insulin Dependant Diabetic Patients', *Am. J. Clin. Nutr.*, 34:184-190 (1981). Data from Jenkins, D., et al., 'The Glycaemic Response to Carbohydrate Foods', *Lancet*, 2:388-391 (1984) and Jenkins, D. et al., 'Diabetic Diets and Carbohydrate Digestibility', Diabetologia, 23:477-484 (1983).
52. Jan Ziegler, 'A Sweet Spice for Diabetics: Cinnamon may Boost the Effects of Insulin', *American Health*, November 1989; summarizes USDA Human Nutrition Research Center in vitro study showing cinnamon, cloves, turmeric and bay leaves tripled insulin action.
53. The Swannanoa Health Report, 1988, 1:1, PO Box 348, Ivy VA 22945
54. L. Griffin, *Insulin vs. Herbs*, Hawkes Publishing, Salt Lake City UT, 1977
55. R. Large et al., 'A Hypoglycaemic Substance from the Roots of the Devil's Club (Fatsia Horrida)', *The Canadian Medical Association Journal*, July 1938, pp. 32-35
56. *Annals of the New York Academy of Sciences*, 447:389- 392 (1985)
57. A. Houtsmuller et al., 'Favourable Influences of Linoleic Acid on the Progression of Diabetic Micro- and Macroangiopathy', *Nutr. Metab.* 24(Suppl.1): 105-118 (1980); A.J. Houtsmuller et al., 'Favourable Influences of Linoleic Acid on the Progression of Diabetic Micro- and Macroangiopathy in Adult Onset Diabetes Mellitus', *Prog. Lipids Research* 20:377-386 (1982).
58. *Omega-6 Essential Fatty Acids: Pathophysiology and Roles in Clinical Medicine*, ed. D.F. Horrobin, Wiley-Liss, 1990. Page 29 shows the plasma phospholipid levels of LA and its major metabolites from diabetic neuropathy cases. LA is above normal, GLA well below and DGLA at about 75% of normal, while AA is about 80% of normal. Evening primrose oil boosts all derivatives and actually normalizes DGLA, and this is associated with prevention and/or regression of diabetic neuropathy. Four chapters are devoted to evening primrose oil effects in diabetes.
59. P. Watkins, (letter), *New England Journal of Medicine*, 12 April 1990, 322(15):1078-9.
60. K. West, 'Diet Therapy for Diabetes: An Analysis of Failure', *Annals of Internal Medicine*, 79:425-434 (1973)
61. L. Sacca et al., 'Insulin Antagonistic Effects of Epinephrine and Glucagon in the Dog', *Am. J. Physiology*, 237(6):E487-E492 (1979)
62. W. Pierpaoli et al., 'Melatonin: a Principal Neuro Immunoregulatory and Anti-Stress Hormone: its Anti-Ageing Effect', *Immunology Letters*, 16:350-362

63. J.R. Samples, 'Effect of Melatonin on Intra-Ocular Pressure', *Current Eye Research*, 7(7):649-53 (1988)
64. K. McAuliffe, 'Live 20 Years Longer, Look 20 Years Younger', *Longevity*, October 1990
65. J.M. Fontenot, 'Melatonin Deficiency: Its Role in Oncogenesis and Age-Related Pathology', *J. Orthomolecular Medicine*, 5(1):22-4 (1990)
66. 'Searching for a Better Pill', *Newsweek*, 8 April, 1991
67. G. Maestroni et al., 'Role of the Pineal Gland in Immunity. Melatonin Antagonizes the Immuno-Suppressive Effects of Acute Stress via an Opiatergic Mechanism', *Immunology*, 63:465-469
68. C.S. Moy et al., *Circulation*, July, 1990
69. M. Mayall, 'Beating the Sugar Blues', *East West Journal*, September 1983
70. D. Davies et al., 'Food Antibodies and Myocardial Infarction', *Lancet*, 25 May 1984, pp. 1012-1014.
71. M. Smith et al., 'Food Intolerance, Atopy and Irritable Bowel Syndrome', *Lancet*, 9 November 1985, p. 1064. 28 IBS patients were predominantly atopic (60%), and 9 improved when they avoided certain foods.
72. A. Wright et al., 'Food Allergy or Intolerance in Severe Recurrent Aphthous Ulceration in the Mouth', *Br. Med. J.*, 292:1237 (1986).
73. ' "Food Allergy": Fact or Fiction', *Lancet*, 25 February 1978, pp. 426-427.
74. J. Eggar et al., 'Is Migraine Food Allergy?', *Lancet*, ii:865-869 (1983)
75. G. Cohen et al. 'Severe Anemia and Chronic Bronchitis Associated With a Markedly Elevated Specific IgG to Cow's Milk Protein', *Annals of Allergy*, 55:38-40 (1985)
76. A. Parke et al., 'Rheumatoid Arthritis and Food: A Case Study', *Br. Med. J.*, 282:2027-2029, (1981)
77. C. Little et al., 'Platelet Serotonin Release in Rheumatoid Arthritis: A Study in Food intolerant Patients', *Lancet*, 6 August 1983, pp. 297-299.
78. J. Gerrard, 'Food Intolerance', *Lancet*, 18 August 1984, pp. 413-414.
79. T. Nsouli, *Pediatric News*, 25(2), (1991)
80. J. Douglass, 'Hygienic Management of Hypertension', *The Western Journal of Medicine*, 142(3):402-403 (1985)
81. R. MacDougall, *My Fight Against Multiple Sclerosis*. MacDougall, London, 1975
82. A. Coca, *The Pulse Test*. Lyle Stuart, Secaucus NJ, 1982, pp. 149-151
83. J. Graham, *Multiple Sclerosis*. Healing Arts Press, Rochester VT, 1989, Ch. 9
84. A. Cant et al., 'Food Hypersensitivity Made Life Threatening by Ingestion of Aspirin', *Br. Med. J.*, 288:755-756 (1984)
85. J. Bienenstock, 'Mucosal Barrier Functions', *Nutrition Reviews*, 42(3):105-108 (1984)
86. R. Cathcart, 'The Vitamin C Treatment of Allergy and the Normally Unprimed State of Antibodies', *Medical Hypotheses*, 21(3):307-321 (1986)
87. C. Ortolani et al., 'Prophylaxis of Adverse Reactions to Foods. A Double-Blind Study of Oral Sodium Cromoglycate for the Prophylaxis of Adverse Reactions to Foods and Additives', *Annals of Allergy*, 50:105-109 (1983)
88. H. Sinclair, 'Deficiency of Essential Fatty Acids and Atherosclerosis, Etcetera', *Lancet*, 7 April 1956, pp. 381-383
89. D.F. Horrobin, 'The Lowering of Plasma Cholesterol Levels by Essential

Fatty Acids', in *Clinical Uses of Essential Fatty Acids*, ed. D.F. Horrobin, Eden Press, Canada, 1982
90. J. Raloff, 'Do You Know Your HDL?', *Science News*, 136(11):171-173 (1989)
91. J. Raloff, 'Do You Know Your HDL?', *Science News*, 136(11):171-173 (1989)
92. *Physicians' Desk Reference*, Medical Economics, Oradell NJ, 1987
93. B. Liebman, 'The HDL/Triglycerides Trap', *Nutrition Action*, 17(7):5-7 (1990)
94. J.D. Hubbard et al., 'Nathan Pritikin's Heart', *New England J. of Med.*, July 4, 1985
95. Data from R. Stallones, 'The Rise and Fall of Ischemic Heart Disease', *Scientific American*, 243(5):53-59 (1980), J. Booyens, 'The Eskimo Diet'. See next reference. *Medical Hypotheses*, 21:387-408 (1986) and other sources.
96. J. Booyens and C. Louwrens, 'The Eskimo Diet. Prophylactic Effects Ascribed to the Balanced Presence of Natural "cis" Unsaturated Essential Fatty Acids and the Absence of Unnatural "trans" and "cis" Isomers of Essential Fatty Acids', *Medical Hypotheses*, 21:387-408 (1986)
97. R. Stallones, 'The Rise and Fall of Ischemic Heart Disease', *Scientific American*, 243(5):53-59 (November 1980)
98. R. Gilchrist, 'Edinburgh Tradition in Clinical Cardiology', *Scottish Med. J.*, 17:284 (1972)
99. R. Mensink et al., 'Effect of Dietary trans Fatty Acids on High-Density and Low-Density Lipoprotein Cholesterol Levels in Healthy Subjects', *New England Journal of Medicine*, 323(7):439-445 (1990)
100. L. Thomas et al., 'Ischemic Heart Disease and the Proportions of Hydrogenated Fat and Ruminant-Animal Fat in Adipose Tissue at Post-Mortem Examination: A Case-Control Study', *J. Epidemiology and Community Health*, 35:251-255 (1981)
101. Leo H. Thomas et al., 'Concentration of 18:1 and 16:1 transunsaturated Fatty Acids in the Adipose Tissue of Decendents Dying of Ischemic Heart Disease Compared with Controls', *Journal of Epidemiology and Community Health*, 37:16-24 (1983)
102. J. Booyens, 'Atherogenesis. An Epidemiological Model Based on the Presence of Unnatural trans and cis Isomers of Unsaturated Fatty Acids in the Maternal Diet and in Mothers' Milk', *Medical Hypotheses*, 21(3):323-333 (1986)
103. M.F. Oliver, 'Fats and Atheroma', *British Medical Journal*, 31 March 1979
104. D. Horrobin, 'A New Concept of Lifestyle-Related Cardiovascular Disease: The Importance of Interactions Between Cholesterol, Essential Fatty Acids, Prostaglandin E1 and Thromboxane A2', *Medical Hypotheses*, 6:785-800 (1980)
105. D. Kromhout et al., 'The Inverse Relation Between Fish Consumption and 20-year Mortality from Coronary Heart Disease', *New England Journal of Medicine*, 312:1205-1209 (1985)
106. A. Leaf and P.C. Webber, 'Cardiovascular Effects of the n-3 Fatty Acids', *New Eng. J. Med.*, 318(9):549-557 (1988)
107. 'Fish Oil Takes a Dive?', *Science News*, 132(22):342 (1987); 'Revealing Finicky Functions of Fish Oil', *Science News*, 135(12):182 (1989).

**108.** G.R. Reis et al., 'Randomized Trial of Fish Oil for Prevention of Restenosis after Coronary Angioplasty', *Lancet*, 22 July 1989
**109.** 'Is Fish Oil a Vitamin Drain?', *Medical Tribune*, 26 April 1987
**110.** Y. Goto, 'Lipid Peroxides as a Cause of Vascular Disease' in K. Yagi, ed., *Lipid Peroxides in Biology And Medicine*, Academic Press, New York, 1982
**111.** 'Prostyacyclin and Atherosclerosis', *Human Pathology*, 16(3):201 (1985)
**112.** R. Saynor and F. Ryan, *The Eskimo Diet*. Ebury Press, London, 1990
**113.** J.R. Beetens et al., 'Influence of Vitamin C on the Metabolism of Arachidonic Acid and the Development of Aortic Lesions during Experimental Atherosclerosis in Rabbits', *Biochem. Biochim. Acta* 43:S274-S276 (1984); 'Prostacyclin and Atherosclerosis', *Human Pathology*, 16(3):210
**114.** J. Raloff, 'Vitamin C Protects Blood From Radicals', *Science News*, 136(9): 133, 1989
**115.** J. Glavind et al., 'The Presence of Peroxidized Lipids in the Atherosclerotic Aorta', *Acta Path.*, 30(1):1 (1951); 'Angiotoxicity of Oxygenated Sterols and Possible Precursors', *Science*, 207:651 (1980); Y. Goto, 'Lipid Peroxides as a Cause of Vascular Disease', K. Yagi, ed., *Lipid Peroxides in Biology and Medicine*, Academic Press, 1982; etc.
**116.** C. Spittle, 'Atherosclerosis and Vitamin C', *Lancet*, 11 December 1971, p. 1280; 'Vitamin C and Myocardial Infarction', *Lancet*, 31 October 1979, p. 931
**117.** This interim result of the Physician's Health Study was announced at the American Heart Association conference in Dallas on Tuesday, 13 November 1990
**118.** S. Rashad, 'Effect of Non-Steroidal Anti-Inflammatory Drugs on the Course of Osteoarthritis', *Lancet*, 2 September 1989, pp. 519-522
**119.** P. Oster et al., 'Blood Pressure and Adipose Tissue Linoleic Acid', *Res. Exp. Med.*, 175:287-291 (1979)
**120.** E. Berry et al., 'Does Dietary Linoleic Acid Influence Blood Pressure?', *Am. J. Clin. Nutr.*, 44:336- 340 (1986)
**121.** as above reference.
**122.** A. Leeds, 'Effects of n-6 Essential Fatty Acids as Evening Primrose Oil in Mild Hypertension', in D. Horrobin, ed., *Omega-6 Essential Fatty Acids*, Wiley-Liss, NY, 1990
**123.** C.P. Venter et al., 'Effects of Essential Fatty Acids on Mild to Moderate Essential Hypertension', *Prostaglandins, Leukotrienes and Essential Fatty Acids*, 33:49-51 (1988)
**124.** D. Mills et al., 'Dietary n-6 and n-3 Fatty Acids and Stress-Induced Hypertension', in D. Horrobin, ed., *Omega-6 Essential Fatty Acid*, Wiley-Liss, NY, 1990
**125.** 'Vitamin C May Reduce Hypertension Risk', *Science News*, 137(19):292 (1990)
**126.** J. Douglass et al., 'Obesity Regimen', *Medical Tribune*, 25 January 1984, 25:30
**127.** J. Douglass et al., 'Effects of a Raw Food Diet on Hypertension and Obesity', *Southern Medical Journal*, 78(7):841-844 (1985)
**128.** E. Mitchel et al., 'Clinical Characteristics and Serum Essential Fatty Acid Levels in Hyperactive Children', *Clin. Paediatr*, 0:406-411 (1987)

**129.** M. Aman et al., 'The Effects of Essential Fatty Acid Supplementation by *Efamol* in Hyperactive Children', *J. Abnorm. Child Psych.*, 15:75-90 (1987); E. Arnold, 'Gamma-Linolenic Acid for Attention Deficit Disorder: Placebo-Controlled Comparison to Amphetamine', Am. Acad. Child. Adolescent Psychiatry, Annual Meeting, Washington DC (1987)
**130.** M. Blackburn, 'Use of *Efamol* (Oil of Evening Primrose) for Depression and Hyperactivity in Children', in D. Horrobin, ed., *Clinical Uses of the Essential Fatty Acids*, Eden Press, Montreal, 1982
**131.** S. Levine, 'Selenium and Human Chemical Hypersensitivities: Preliminary Findings', *Int. J. Biosocial Res.*, 3(1):44-47 (1982); 'Oxidants/Anti-Oxidants and Chemical Hypersensitivities I', *Int. J. Biosocial Res.*, 4(1):51-54 (1983); 'Oxidants/Anti-Oxidants and Chemical Hypersensitivities II', *Int. J. Biosocial Res.*, 4(2):102-105 (1983)
**132.** D. Horrobin, 'Use of Evening Primrose Oil (*Efamol*) In Psychiatric Disorders', *Efamol* Research Institute.
**133.** Y. Abdullah et al., 'Effect of ADP on PGE Formation in Blood Platelets from Patients with Depression, Mania and Schizophrenia', *British Journal of Psychiatry*, 127:591-595 (1975)
**134.** D. Horrobin and J. Lieb, 'A Biochemical Basis for the Actions of Lithium on Behaviour and Immunity: Relapsing and Remitting Disorders of Inflammation and Immunity such as Multiple Sclerosis or Recurrent Herpes as Manic-Depression of the Immune System', *Medical Hypotheses*, 7:891-905 (1981)
**135.** A. Voors, 'Lithium Depletion and Atherosclerotic Heart Disease', *Lancet*, 2:670 (1970)
**136.** S. Nasr et al., 'Coincidental Improvement in Asthma during Lithium Treatment', *Am. J. Psych.*, 134:1042-1043 (1977)
**137.** J. Reiffers et al., 'Cutaneous Side-Effects of Lithium', *Dermatologica*, 155:155-163 (1977); G. Christodoulu et al., 'Positive Side-Effects of Lithium', *Am. J. Psych.*, 135:1249 (1978)
**138.** J. Lieb, 'Linoleic Acid in the Treatment of Lithium Toxicity and Familial Tremor', *Prosta. Med.*, 4:275-279 (1980)
**139.** H. Sinclair, 'History of the Essential Fatty Acids', in D. Horrobin, ed., *Omega-6 Essential Fatty Acids*, Wiley-Liss, New York, 1990
**140.** D. Horrobin, 'Loss of Delta-6-Desaturase Activity as a Key Factor in Ageing', *Medical Hypotheses*, 7:1211-1220, 1981
**141.** 'More Overweight in Spite of Healthy Eating Campaigns', *The Times*, 15 June 1990, p. 5
**142.** P. Oster et al., 'Linoleic Acid and Blood Pressure', *Prog. Fd. Nutr. Sci.*, 4(5):39-40 (1980)
**143.** A.E. Hansen, 'Role of Unsaturated Dietary Fat in Infant Nutrition', *Am. J. Pub. Health*, 47:1367-1370 (1957); A.E. Hansen et al., 'Essential Fatty Acids in Human Nutrition', *J. Nutr.*, 60:565-576 (1958)
**144.** N.J. Rothwell et al., 'A Role for Brown Adipose Tissue in Diet-Induced Thermogenesis', *Nature*, 281:31-35 (1979)
**145.** J. Heaton, 'The Distribution of Brown Adipose Tissue in the Human', *J. Anatomy*, 112:35-39 (1972)
**146.** R.H. Llowndes and R.E. Mansel, 'The Effects of Evening Primrose Oil Administration on the Serum Lipids of Normal and Obese Human Subjects',

in D. Horrobin, ed., *Clinical Uses of the Essential Fatty Acids*, Eden Press, Montreal, 1982

147. K. Vaddaddi and D. Horrobin, 'Weight Loss Produced by Evening Primrose Oil Administration in Normal and Schizophrenic Subjects', *IRCS J. Med. Sci.*, 7:52 (1979); M. Mir et al., 'The Effects of Evening Primrose Oil (*Efamol*) on Erythrocyte Sodium Transport and Obesity', in D. Horrobin, ed., *Clinical Uses of the Essential Fatty Acids*, Eden Press, Montreal, 1982
148. G. Bray, *Canadian Standardized Test of Fitness*, 1986
149. 'Arthritic Origins in the New World?', *Science News*, 133(15):232 (1988)
150. S. Rashad, 'Effect of Non-Steroidal Anti-Inflammatory Drugs on the Course of Osteoarthritis', *Lancet*, 2 September 1989, pp. 519-522
151. J. Belch et al., 'The Effect of Evening Primrose Oil (EPO) and EPO/Fish Oil Combination on Rheumatoid Arthritis: A Double Blind Study', *Br. J. Rheumatism*, 25:2 Abs. 75 (1986)
152. J. Mulinare et al., 'Periconceptual Use of Multivitamins and the Occurrence of Neural Tube Defects', *JAMA*, 260(21):3141-3145 (1988)
153. D. Benton, 'Effect of Vitamin and Mineral Supplementation on Intelligence of a Sample of Schoolchildren', *Lancet*, 23 January 1988, pp. 140-143
154. S. Schonenthaler, 'The Impact of a Low Food Additive and Sucrose Diet on Academic Performance in 803 New York City Public Schools', *Intl. J. Biosocial Res.*, 8(2):185-195 (1986)
155. R. Beach et al., 'Gestational Zinc Deprivation in Mice: Persistence of Immunodeficiency for Three Generations', *Science*, 218:469-471, 1982
156. J. Raloff, 'Does Foetal Zinc Affect Later Immunity?', *Science News*, 131(24):375, 1987
157. 'Pregnancy Hypertension Marker Found', *Science News*, 131(22):344, 1987
158. E. Alder et al., 'Breast-Feeding and Post Natal Depression', *J. Psychosom. Res.*, 27:139-144 (1983)
159. J.K. Pye et al., 'Clinical Experience of Drug Treatment for Mastalgia', *Lancet*, 17 August 1985, pp. 373-376
160. 'Pay Offs', *Financial Mail*, 8 June 1990

# Index